Breaking Little Bones

Breaking
Little Bones

triumph and trauma, the first cures of childhood leukemia

G. BENNETT HUMPHREY

G. Bennett.Humphrey@gmail.com

Published

ISBN 099770280X
ISBN 13: 9780997702804

Contents

Preface

"This is a long-awaited homage to saints and soldiers. This is a story of children, parents, and doctors brought together by Providence to travel a path together that led to cures for childhood leukemia. Yes, it is a book about tragedies and sadness, but, it is also a book that you won't be able to put down, nor will you forget the experiences it will bring to you. Humanity wins. You will forever remember the image of courageous little saints who met each difficulty by wiping their mouths with the back of their hands and moving forward. Their courage and indefatigability inspired the compassion and dedication of many physicians and nurses who fought until they won. Our family is so grateful that these saints and soldiers made this journey."

Grace Dowling Afridi
Parent of a leukemia survivor

Advanced Praise and Commentary

"Make no mistake. This is not for the faint of heart. Children of 2 East you come to know and like bring their unique personalities and backgrounds to the field of combat. Some survive and are cured, but most do not. Their stories weave themselves into your consciousness and hold on. Dr. Humphrey succeeds in making the complex world of medicine accessible to the non-professional, and closing the book after the last page leaves you with a sense of quiet triumph."

Rhonda Borders, LCMS, mental health counselor,
and coauthor of *Murder at the Leopard*

"This is a riveting read from start to finish, though not always an easy one. Though this would seem to be a story of failure and heartbreak, it is instead a story of bravery: the bravery of the children, their parents and the medical staff who care for them. There are teddy bears and dogs and wigs and make-up along the way, and amazing as it seems, joy and laughter. This book is well worth reading, for in it Dr. Humphrey brings each child fully to life and we get to meet them, thus giving them the lives they lost. His insight gained along the way is remarkable."

Francie Hall, author of short stories and poetry,
frequent contributor to *Colorado Life* magazine

"Dr. Humphrey has access to an extraordinary world through his caring for young patients, and his concern for them lends his writing authenticity, richness, and generosity."

**Summer Wood, author of *Raising Wrecker*,
recipient of 2012 WILLA Award**

"The vignette structure of Dr. Humphrey's *Breaking Little Bones* works to engage the reader at a deep level of connection without overwhelming him/her, for the subject matter is indeed powerful. The illness and deaths of the children require stamina on the part of the reader as well as Dr. Humphrey. On 2 East, the children's leukemia ward at NIH, Dr. Humphrey is taught by his young patients and their parents about the daily task of living one's ethics and discovering the hues of love. Horses, dogs, squirrels and social activities/dates intersperse our moments on 2 East; levity and ordinary business splice the narrative in vignettes of varying lengths, to delightful effect."

**Annie Dawid, PhD, author of *And Darkness
Was under His Feet: Stories of a Family***

"It's a hugely compelling and tightly focused story, one that's likely to resonate with a broad readership. Well done."

**Justin St. Germain, author of *Son of Gun*,
recipient of Best Book of 2013 at Amazon**

"This is not a mere recital of medical care. It tells the story of how a self-centered scientist becomes a caring physician. The book shows us not only the dignity these dying children display, but the courage and wisdom they show us while they are alive. A great read and engrossing from start to finish."

**Mary Lampe, PhD, historian of Sicily in the Middle
Ages and coauthor of *Murder at the Leopard***

"I really loved it. The book was just wonderful, heart wrenching, and such a great window on a world so few of us (fortunately) see."

Cynthia Storrs, poet, English teacher, Dickinson scholar, and recipient of a National Endowment for the Humanities award

"Dr. Humphrey's introspective reflections on the circumstances and characters of the children of 2 East, their timely and timeless alchemy, offers the reader a window into a young doctor's journey from his head to his heart. I have appreciated the author's willingness to expose the early work on childhood leukemia. His writing reveals the physical and emotional toll it took on the children, parents, and health care providers. Getting it right in medical research is a slow, tedious, and lengthy process of getting it wrong, less wrong and finally making progress. This book is an insightful and engaging story of people whose lives were foundational to the early successes of curing childhood leukemia."

Peggy Godfrey, author, cowboy poet, performer, and former research medical technologist

"Dr. Humphrey shows us the mind of a scientist and the heart of a poet as he guides us through an emotional Olympic event in this multi-faceted account. We share his frustration when directed to follow clinical trial protocols that the associates all find disturbing. Then we are charmed when Todd, a word loving young patient teaches Dr. Humphrey how to pronounce "supercalifragilisticexpialidocious." Every child's death brings deep regret and yet everyone gets on with somber strength and fortitude. Hilarious laughter erupts when almost teenager, Polly checks in for her monthly treatment wearing a T-shirt that says, "Bald is Beautiful. Dr. H is my barber." The doctor dreads inserting the needle to do a bone marrow aspiration. Later, he is filled with a warm presence as he sees three foot tall Walt trudging down the hall, pushing an IV pole, with his little bare bottom peeking out under the hospital gown. A parent never "gets over" the death of a child. We never become our old self again. We can, however, grow into someone with strength, courage, wisdom, and perhaps an ability to comfort others."

Patrician K. Nolan, MEd, poet and author of
***Broken Pieces of Shells*, about the loss of her own son**

"This book may have written for the health care and grief support professions, but all of us can learn from the heart-warming (and heart-breaking) experiences that were so pivotal in the author's year on 2 East."

Pickens Halt, grief counselor and author of
How We Grieve: Regression and Regrowth

Dedication

"That which is done out of love always takes place beyond good and evil."
Friedrich Nietzsche

To Dr. Freireich and others at NIH, who taught
me the importance of clinical research.
To Rick Lottsfeldt and Jerry Sandler, who support-
ed me during my year of transformation.
To the children, mothers, and nurses of 2 East, who ex-
emplified the reciprocal nature of love.

Foreword

Many reviews in scientific journals, as well as best-selling nonfiction books, have been written describing the history of the first cures of cancer. Dr. G. Bennett Humphrey's *Breaking Little Bones* is unique. It's a highly personal, first-hand narrative nonfiction book written from the perspective of a young physician-in-training who treated some of the first children to be cured of acute leukemia. Dr. Humphrey describes in candid detail the conflict he experienced as he became aware that to achieve these seemingly random cures among some of his young patients, other children in his care would die because they were unable to tolerate the intensive chemotherapy that was necessary to eradicate their last leukemic blood cell.

The year was 1964. The location was 2 East, the Pediatric Leukemia Service at the National Institutes of Health (NIH), Bethesda, Maryland, where Dr. Humphrey began a twelve-month assignment as a Commissioned Officer in the US. Public Health Service. The setting was highly challenging, and its heroes—the children with acute leukemia, their moms, and the 2 East nurses—have not been fully appreciated until this personal and candid retrospective. Prior to 1964, acute lymphocytic leukemia was 100 percent fatal. In 1947, Dr. Sidney Farber at the Children's Hospital in Boston had achieved transient remissions treating acute leukemia with antifolic-acid drugs. Dr. Farber's report in the *New England Journal of Medicine* in 1948 established the principle that chemotherapy could have an antileukemic effect and reverse, if only temporarily, the destructive progression of acute leukemia. Shortly thereafter, a team of scientists at NIH, headed by Drs. Emil "Tom" Frei and Emil "Jay" Freireich, pursued the concept that drugs that individually had incomplete antileukemic activity but also caused different toxic effects offered the promise, if combined, of curing acute leukemia. Their first protocols, VAMP (*v*incristine, *a*methoperin, 6-*m*ercaptopurine, *p*rednisone) and BIKE (two cycles), were promising but subject to frequent relapses. The third protocol, POMP (*p*rednisolone, *O*ncovin, *m*ethotrexate and *P*urinethol), was ready to be activated when Drs. Humphrey and Rick Lottsfeldt and I arrived for our tours of duty on 2 East.

Breaking Little Bones describes how we, as three inexperienced, young physicians, still in training, learned that our assignment was not to "protect" our young patients from the toxic effects of chemotherapy but to administer all four drugs in full dose, according to protocol, no matter what else (including infection or low blood counts) was happening. Dr. Humphrey describes his personal struggle as he came to understand that without the full-dose chemotherapy protocol, despite its inevitably toxic and life-threatening side effects, his young patients would not be candidates for the promise of a sustained remission—that is, a cure.

Breaking Little Bones is an insider's perspective of the resilience of these young children in the face of the adversities of their disease and its treatment, the uncompromising love of their mothers, and the professionalism of the 2 East nursing staff. These are the heroes. The villain, acute leukemia, was in retreat, but not without causing heartbreaking pain and suffering. In retrospect, POMP and its designers are also heroes for their groundbreaking progress. Although as Dr. Humphrey notes, it was difficult to recognize that achievement in the heat of the moment.

In 1975, a follow-up survey of sixty-six children who had been treated at NIH with VAMP, BIKE, or POMP protocols determined that ten were still in remission, a cure rate of 15 percent. High-dose combination chemotherapy had achieved its first cures of acute leukemia. However, the limits of this approach to treating leukemia were recognized, and, today, the strategy of treatment-to-cure has shifted to progenitor cell (bone marrow, peripheral blood stem cell, and cord blood) transplantation. Dr. Humphrey's book serves as a permanent record of the vision of the pioneers of NIH's anti-leukemia chemotherapy protocols and the courage of the children on 2 East who made it possible to break through the mind-set that acute leukemia was inevitably fatal.

S. Gerald Sandler, MD, FACP, FCAP
Professor of Medicine and Pathology
Georgetown University Medical Center
Washington, DC

Prelude

"I know something's very, *very* wrong."

"**W**ell, Janice, how's my soccer player doing?" Doctor Fillmore asked.

Janice Polk, a ten-year-old, was normally a happy, talkative kid, but this morning, she sat close to her mother and didn't respond. So her mother said, "We're not doing so well. Janice just hasn't been herself; she lacks energy. Last night, she felt warm, so I took her temperature. It was ninety-nine."

Doctor Fillmore went through a child's infectious-disease physical exam: Is the skin free of any rashes? Any sounds in the chest? Is the abdomen soft? Are the eardrums red? Is there a white exudate in the back of the throat? And finally, is the neck supple, and are there any swollen lymph nodes?

"I didn't find anything, Mrs. Polk. It's probably a low-grade infection. I'll put her on an antibiotic; she should feel better in a day or two."

Three days later, Mrs. Polk and Janice were back in the office. "Janice isn't better—if anything, a little worse. She just wants to stay inside. I'm sorry, but I'm worried."

Doctor Fillmore repeated his exam. He paused and said the antibiotic he had chosen, a tetracycline, was good, but he wanted Janice on something stronger. "It's called chloramphenicol."

Two days later, Mrs. Polk and Janice were in the office for an early first appointment. "I know: something is very, *very* wrong, Doctor. Janice hasn't wanted to get out of bed, and this morning, I noticed these little red dots on her skin, and her tummy is enlarged. I didn't sleep at all last night. I'm worried."

After examining every inch of Janice's skin, Doctor Fillmore excused himself and said he'd be right back. On returning he said, "I'm referring Janice to a pediatrician, John Kent. His office is right next to the hospital here in Fairfax, and he'll see her this morning, just as soon as you can get there. You'll like him; he's a nice guy."

Fairfax, Virginia, wasn't a very large city, so it was a short drive. "A specialist, a children's doctor. Well, at least he isn't a surgeon," Mrs. Polk thought. She tried to concentrate on the traffic. "But it must be something serious. You can't just get in to see a doctor this fast."

Before they entered the exam room, Doctor Kent explained to the young medical student from Georgetown University who was rotating through his clinic, "This child's been referred as an urgent case by a family doctor, so if you don't mind, we'll see Janice together rather than have you see her first."

Doctor Kent introduced himself and the student first to Janice and then to her mother. He listened to what had happened and asked a few questions. He talked to Janice before he started his exam, telling her what he was going to do and then assuring her, "None of this is going to hurt." After looking at all of her skin, he gently examined her abdomen, especially the upper region. He explained to Janice, so her mother would understand, that she was going over to the hospital for some tests; it wouldn't take long, and the blood work would be done within an hour.

Later that morning Doctor Kent said to the student, "We need to discuss Janice's laboratory data. This is an important teaching case but a tragic state of affairs. Look at these lab slips. Janice has bone-marrow failure due to leukemia. She's anemic. There are no normal white blood cells—only leukemic blasts. Her platelets are very low; those skin lesions are petechiae. Her slightly distended abdomen is due to leukemic infiltration of the spleen and liver. It all fits."

"But why the prescriptions of antibiotics?" the student asked.

"It's a common practice. Viral infections are very common, and antibiotics are not indicated. But many parents will want some sort of treatment. Physicians know the fastest way to manage a case is an unnecessary course of an antibiotic. It takes time to explain to parents that observation is the best course of action."

"Shouldn't Doctor Fillmore have ordered lab tests on the first or second visit?"

"Good question. That's what you're going to learn during your pediatrics residency. If he had felt an enlarged spleen—yes. If he really thought she could have a bacterial infection—yes. Fillmore's not a bad doc, and he always refers if he's in trouble. Well, let's go see Mrs. Polk. These disclosures are never easy on anyone—mother, child, family members, or me."

Mrs. Polk was taken into an examining room while one of the doctor's staff entertained Janice in the office's playroom.

Doctor Kent and the student entered the room and sat down. Doctor Kent had smiled while talking to Janice. Now the smile was gone. "The problem, Mrs. Polk, is in Janice's blood. I'm sorry. The tests show that she has leukemia."

"Oh, no. No—no." Tears streamed down her cheeks. With a trembling hand, she accepted a tissue. "I just knew that it was something bad." She wiped away tears. "Something terrible."

He waited and then explained, "Leukemia is a disease of the bone marrow that interrupts the production of healthy blood cells. Janice is anemic; that's why she's been inactive. The leukemia has enlarged her liver and spleen, and that was why her stomach is enlarged. Her marrow no longer makes a little particle that controls bleeding. The little red dots on her skin are small hemorrhages. On seeing those red spots, Doctor Fillmore was right to call me and request that Janice be seen right away."

Again he waited until she looked up. He explained that he had made arrangements for Janice to be admitted to the Clinical Center at NIH over in Bethesda.

Mrs. Polk sniffled. "Why there? I thought those were all research buildings."

"NIH has been interested in leukemia for a number of years. There is even a special ward just for children. It's called 2 East. I've heard the head of the unit speak. His name is Freireich, but Janice will be cared for by one of his young clinical associates. They have—"

"Who are these young doctors? Are they medical students?"

"Doctor Freireich's clinical associates have all finished medical school. They're all MDs who have also finished an internship and a residency. Young physicians from all over the country come to learn more about leukemia on 2 East so they can specialize in oncology." After a short pause, he added, "Would you like us to call someone to drive you over to NIH?"

"No. Thanks. I'm OK." She sighed. "I've been going through hell not knowing. Now I know. This is a different kind of hell. Leukemia. I'll be OK."

So on an overcast day in April 1965, Mrs. Polk pulled into the visitors' parking lot next to the Clinical Center. Her mind was full of words, short phrases, and incomplete sentences. "Leukemia. Now we know… Why would a doctor want to study leukemia…? 2 East. My daughter… this bad, bad, disease…"

As Janice got out of the car, she whined, "Not another doctor."

"Yes, dear, we'll just have to see what this one is like, won't we?"

As Mrs. Polk entered 2 East, she hesitated and said to herself, "I wonder who our new doctor is going to be."

Part I:
The Learning Curve

JULY

First week

July 1, 1964. As I stood before a door labeled "2 East, Children's Leukemia Ward, National Cancer Institute," I set my shoulders. Humphrey, I thought, you're an internist. What the hell are you doing here?

Pediatrics. An internist asking a one-year-old infant, "Where does it hurt?" wasn't a very bright idea. Telling a crying three-year-old there wasn't anything to be frightened of wasn't likely to work either. How was I going to manage?

During the past year, as a PhD. postdoctoral fellow, I worked in a research laboratory in Mainz, Germany; I was spontaneous and not self-conscious about my manner. But now, walking through that 2 East door, I had to wear the persona of a physician.

I told myself, "March!" I was, after all, an officer. Which persona would be appropriate? I could try to look like an overconfident diagnostician. Or I could pretend to be the relaxed, know-it-all physician. How about the persona of I'm-anxious-to-get-started doctor? I opened the door and presented myself.

More like a trench than a hospital ward, 2 East was a long dark hall. The walls were painted gun-barrel gray green and the linoleum floor a mismatched gray black. Halfway down the hall was a brightly lit nurses' station, the command post of 2 East. A nurse walked out of the station toward me. She wore a standard white one-piece knee-length uniform. A nurse's cap was perched neatly on short black hair.

3

"Good morning, I'm Dee, the head nurse here on 2 East. You must be one of our new clinical associates." Her manner was professional but cordial.

I mustered a facade of confidence. "I'm Doctor Humphrey."

"Last year's clinical associates are in the playroom with three of my staff. It's the second room on your left." Like a good shepherd, Dee led me down the hall and opened the door.

I thanked her and walked in.

"Good morning. I'm Ben Humphrey, assigned to this unit."

A young man stepped forward. "John Billingsworth. You're taking over my cases."

He ignored my extended hand and pointed to three charts. I suggested we see the patients together.

"Not necessary. It's all in my notes," he said, "or on the pillowcase." He shook his head. "You're going to love giving POMP to these kids." Without another word, he was gone.

"Come on, Doctor H., I'll take you around and introduce you to your kids," a nurse said.

"Thank you." I didn't notice her name tag, face, or figure because my mind was on meeting three pediatric patients. An internist might not want to admit he was scared of a toddler, but he could afford to acknowledge some trepidation.

"Don't be too critical of Doctor B," she said. "His one-year tour of duty on 2 East is now over."

In the first room, a three-year-old boy sat among a zoo of stuffed animals. He appeared in no distress—apparently indifferent to the dried blood covering his face and hands. He clutched a teddy bear also coated with blood.

"Billy Sullivan has leukemia, and he's is in remission," the nurse said, handing me the chart. "He finished a course of POMP ten days ago and now has a very low platelet count. Billy was admitted this morning with an actively bleeding nose. Doctor B ordered a platelet transfusion;

one of the physicians from Ear, Nose, and Throat will pack his nose this morning."

The pillowcase was red.

Billy offered me his bloodstained teddy bear. I took it, pretended to examine the abdomen, and returned the bear with a smile. He smiled back. In the past, as an internist, I was often given a bottle of booze by a grateful patient. Now a child had trusted me with his most prized possession. The nurse told me that not everybody was allowed to hold that bear.

In the second room, a quiet eleven-year-old boy lay on his back, his nasogastric tube hooked up to a suction pump. A stack of four books stood on his bedside table. He didn't move as we walked in. Even an internist didn't have to ask if he was in pain.

"John Graham has an abdominal lymphoma and receives radiation therapy."

I interrupted her: "He has bowel obstruction."

A green patch of bile stained the pillowcase. The bowel obstruction had forced bilious secretions from the duodenum back up into the stomach. When I asked John if he could point to any pain, he shook his head. With a light touch, not a real palpation, I performed the ritual laying on of the hands. There was a fullness and slight distension of his abdomen. The diagnosis of obstruction of the small bowel had been established, and he was receiving therapy to shrink the tumor.

In the third room, a six-year-old girl sat on the edge of her bed playing with a doll. She noted our entrance, did not smile, and continued dressing her doll.

"Sarah Thompkins is in remission and receives monthly POMP. It makes most of them sick to their stomach. They hate it."

Vomited cereal spattered the pillowcase.

After a glance, she continued combing her doll's hair. Sarah allowed me to palpate her abdomen; there was no enlargement of the spleen. She was cooperative and polite, didn't smile, and just wanted me to leave. She wasn't going to pretend to like me. How honest and refreshing. We respected her wish and returned to the nurses' station.

"For the moment, everything is OK, Doctor Humphrey. The chemotherapy orders for this week were written yesterday. Why don't you take a break? I'm sure you'd like to meet the other two associates."

"Thank you for introducing me to my patients. What are the visiting hours for parents?"

"This afternoon you'll have an opportunity to meet the kids' mothers."

Her name tag read "Morgan." A short, peppy, attractive young woman, she had touched each child on the shoulder while introducing me.

"Do you enjoy working on the unit?"

"Oh yes. I asked to be assigned here. In a pediatrician's office, it's chart work and shots. Not why I went into nursing."

I frowned and cocked my head to one side. "Then you're not a commissioned officer in the Public Health Service assigned to 2 East?"

"Nope. No one has to salute me," Morgan said with a smile.

I didn't go into medicine to watch toddlers die, flashed through my mind. I elected not to share that thought with her.

"Well, if you'll excuse me, I need to change some pillowcases."

Morgan had educated me about a couple of minor toxicities, and she had a nice way with my patients. She had made the morning a pleasant encounter by putting me at ease. If I needed to know something, I'd just ask Morgan.

• • •

While the other two clinical associates finished their introductory rounds, I waited in the doctors' office. The wall and floor of the office were the same drab colors as the hall. A two-year-old telephone book sat on the second shelf of the bookcase. Each of the three metal desks had a phone. A new 1964 telephone directory for NIH had been placed on each desk.

The other two associates entered the office. We exchanged basic background information: where we went to medical school, type of residency, any postresidency training. Facts for potential ranking in a pecking order.

"Rick Lottsfeldt, University of Washington for med school and pediatrics. Fellowship in hematology and oncology in Minnesota."

"Jerry Sandler, NYU–Bellevue for both med school and residency in internal medicine." Jerry reached out and shook our hands.

"Ben Humphrey, med school and residency in medicine, University of Chicago; last year I worked in a research laboratory in Mainz, Germany."

Rick was the tallest of the three of us, his ample head of brown hair sat in disarray on his head, and his very easy manner reminded me of Andy Griffith. Jerry was the shortest and slightly stocky, his pitch-black hair had a slight wave, and his warm outgoing manner reminded me of Tony Bennett. I was six feet tall and very thin, my short black hair was combed into place, and I tended to be polite and reserved when meeting people.

We sat together. Rick seemed at ease, a pediatrician on a pediatric floor. Jerry yakked about something. He liked to talk. I pretended not to be scared. The greater my fear, the less I had to say.

"Uh, you guys are internists. If I were assigned to an adult nursing unit, I'd need help," Rick said.

"Well, you've got that right. Bellevue didn't prepare me for this."

"As a resident in Chicago, I never set foot on a pediatric floor," I chimed in.

Rick opened his hands. "If you two have any questions about taking care of your kids, please ask me or call me at home anytime—but I don't mean to interfere."

Jerry and I looked at each other.

"Thanks. I appreciate that," Jerry said.

"I'm going to need all the help I can get."

No reason for us not to be friends. I didn't expect any antagonism either, especially after Rick's remark and Jerry admitting he'd accept Rick's help.

Vietnam was a real threat to young physicians; that was why we had competed for a post at NIH. During wars, friendships are forged under fire watching friends die. Our friendship would be forged on this nursing unit, under fire from the senior staff, and the friends we'd watch die were the children of 2 East.

• • •

How was I going to survive? A sinking feeling weighted on my chest. Death from leukemia couldn't be prevented, but I didn't want anybody dying because I missed something.

I had no intention of pretending I knew anything about children. If I recognized a problem, I would ask for help. If someone thought my question stupid, I couldn't care less. Good patient care came first. A dumb question might tarnish my reputation, but my ego could handle that.

This would be my first experience of unattended work rounds. I had gained my clinical expertise in internal medicine on daily team rounds. Every morning, two medical students, two interns, and at least one resident reviewed the status of all of our patients. We discussed real or potential problems on faculty-conducted teaching rounds three times per week. On 2 East, I'd make rounds several times a day, always alone. Once a week, we'd make rounds with a senior staff member.

Here, I felt as uneasy as the first night in 1960 I took call as an intern.

• • •

At a quarter to noon, I bought a cup of coffee on the first floor of the Clinical Center and crossed the street to a bench near a large tree. After I shared the last corner of my sandwich with a squirrel, I walked. The campus of NIH rested on low rolling hills. Most of the thirty-one red brick buildings were low. Lawns and trees separated the buildings, curved streets, and sidewalks, inviting one to roam.

As I walked, I thought, what do you know that might help this afternoon? I did know something about POMP. The National Cancer Institute (NCI) staff had sent me the POMP protocol, which I read several times during my last few weeks in Germany. Therapy consisted of five days of intravenous drugs known to be effective treating leukemia. These were prednisolone, Oncovin or vincristine, methotrexate, and Purinethol or 6-mercaptopurine. This schedule often caused toxicity, fevers, infections, bleeding, and vomiting—to mention only a few troublesome side effects. On rounds this morning, I had observed two minor toxicities: bleeding and vomiting. Major toxicities, such as overwhelming bacterial infections, could be life-threatening or even fatal.

You know a lot about leukemia and lymphomas, I told myself. My dissertation was on a mouse model of leukemia. When the origin of the leukemogenic event is in the bone marrow, the cells readily enter the blood and invade every organ. When the malignancy starts in a lymph node, it's a solid mass of tissue that can cause obstruction in the surrounding tissues and is referred to as a lymphoma.

• • •

I remembered Morgan's statement, "You'll have an opportunity to meet the mothers." To me, that wasn't an opportunity; it was a threat. The last time I had touched a child was as a junior med student in 1958. I worried about getting through the year, but now my concern focused on rounds with mothers this afternoon.

Mothers! What did I know about mothers? Nothing. For me as an internist, a mother was a caring adult having years of experience with a pediatric person. A knowledgeable woman who could understand an illiterate infant's needs, whose day was filled with interruptions and dirty diapers, and who for some inexplicable reason wasn't an alcoholic. This mature female had successfully completed years of childhood care and would now look to me to treat her son or daughter. For the next few weeks, the way to approach the mothers of 2 East was going to lie in honesty, not knowledge.

Mothers didn't want to turn the care of their son or daughter over to an inexperienced doctor, and I had no experience in three critical areas: pediatrics, leukemia in humans, and the drugs used in the POMP protocol. How would I deal with my lack of knowledge?

Doctor Billingsworth had written excellent off-service notes in each chart recording the date of diagnosis, response to POMP, number of courses, and any complications. I would take the patient's chart into each room and, after a few cordial remarks to the mother and patient, sit down and review the information; then I would ask the mother if there was anything else I ought to know. Then I would assure her I'd find the answers to any questions she might have.

Before my afternoon rounds, Morgan told me, "We asked the mothers to start their daily visits this afternoon so the new doctors could get acquainted with their patients."

The nurses might have known that two of three doctors were internists, but the mothers knew nothing. "The mothers are eager to meet you; they're also apprehensive. They've gotten used to last year's clinical associates," Morgan said.

As a resident in internal medicine, I was assigned to a subspecialty service for three months. The interns rotated every month. So there would be a new intern each month, and some patients could be quite outspoken in their opinions of the new physician. While they got used to their new intern in a few days, the initial comments were almost always negative. I understood that, for a period of time, I wouldn't be as good as Doctor Billingsworth.

• • •

I started my rounds at two o'clock. Mrs. Graham held a book so her son, John, could look at a picture of a race car.

"Good afternoon, Doctor Humphrey," Mrs. Graham said. "Won't you please sit down?"

She knew my name.

She wanted to know what universities I had attended and said something positive about the University of Chicago. She commented, "I hope you enjoy living on the East Coast." Then she smoothly changed the subject to her son. "How long before the radiation therapy will reduce the lymphoma to the point that John can eat again? Does radiation therapy cause a granulocytopenia like chemotherapy?"

"I don't want to second-guess the radiation therapists. I'll talk to them this afternoon."

What a warm and intelligent woman. She had asked about "granulocytopenia" rather than using the more common expression "low white-blood-cell count."

In Sarah Thompkins's room, I noticed that the pillowcase and sheets had been changed, and the bed was strewn with doll clothes and a couple of Barbie books. Even I knew Barbie was very popular.

"Good afternoon, Sarah."

Sarah looked at me as she had that morning without responding. I went to the other side of the bed and introduced myself to her mom.

Mrs. Thompkins was thin and short. As she put down her knitting, her hands trembled. She wore a cotton print dress, her hair pulled back in a bun. She searched for the right words before speaking.

"Me and Sarah are pleased to meet you, Doctor."

"Doctor Billingsworth told me about Sarah this morning." That was not exactly true, but I had read Sarah's chart. I reviewed her daughter's progress to date and the current course of POMP. "Do you have any questions, Mrs. Thompkins?"

"No, Doctor."

Mrs. Thompkins put her arm around Sarah's shoulder, and her daughter leaned into her mother's embrace. I decided not to prolong this first encounter beyond thirty minutes.

Mrs. Sullivan and Billy played with a stuffed animal, a monkey. Billy had been cleaned up, the dried blood washed from his face and hands.

His bed was a jumble of stuffed animals, his bloodstained teddy bear tucked under his arm.

Billy looked up at me and smiled. He was receiving an infusion of platelets. Vaseline-soaked gauze strips were packed into each nostril.

"Billy, we'll get back to our story about the monkey, but now I want to meet our new doctor." Mrs. Sullivan turned toward me and said, "You're Doctor Humphrey. Hello."

I smiled; bad news traveled fast on 2 East.

"This is Billy's third nosebleed. Do they always occur a week after therapy?" I asked.

"Yes, that's when his platelet count is the lowest."

She listened to my comments about bleeding, chemotherapy, and a plan for managing Billy's nasal hemorrhage.

She told me, "Thrombocytopenia was less of a threat than fever and infection. It's just part of Billy's therapy."

I frowned.

"Oh, thrombocytopenia? That's what Doctor Billingsworth called it. I liked him, but he had trouble using simple words."

Things on 2 East did not match my expectations. During my residency in medicine, rounds on ten to fifteen patients might take two hours; here on 2 East, two hours had been spent with three patients and their mothers. The physical exam on an adult during rounds was limited to the area of the body that was infirm, the abdomen on Gastroenterology, the heart on Cardiology, and so on. This afternoon, I elected to do a complete exam in front of the mother. The adult team tried not to act hurried when talking to a patient, but time was always short, and the team remained standing while in the patient's room. Now I was sitting down, taking time to talk and listen. In one afternoon, I became aware of the obvious. Adult patients had relatives. My pediatric patients had something far more important. I would spend this next year being in awe of these young women: mothers.

• • •

I was standing outside the nurses' station when I saw a three-year-old strolling down the hall. Towering over him was a six-foot IV pole on wheels. A bag of fluid hung on the pole, which he pushed with his free hand. He held his other arm, wrapped in gauze taped to a small white board, parallel to the floor. He was taking good care of his IV site. His hospital gown, tied at the shoulders, revealed his little round bare butt.

"Dee, you've got a patient loose in the hall," I said.

She came out of the nurses' station and looked at the boy and then at me, the internist. "Oh, that's Walt, going down to the playroom. He doesn't want any help."

"He's alone!"

She smiled. "We give them all the freedom we can. That's the least we can do."

Hearing his name, Walt turned and flashed a smile.

• • •

After dinner in the cafeteria, I returned to 2 East and reread the POMP protocol. Before leaving the Clinical Center, I went to the nurses' station to ask if there were any problems.

"You're Doctor Humphrey. I'm Barbara, the evening supervisor."

Barbara had snow-white hair and was short, with a solid figure befitting a woman of her age. Although she was probably in her fifties, her demeanor suggested a great deal of reserve energy. Noting my surprise that she knew my name, Barbara explained that Dee had commented on all three new clinical associates. Apparently, the day shift thought we were going to be a good team. Barbara further surprised me when she told me she liked the fact that I had taken Billy Sullivan's bloodstained teddy bear, examined it, and returned it with a smile.

Dumbfounded, I said something about being impressed with my two comrades and then again asked if there were any problems. Barbara assured me that everything was OK. "Why don't you go home, Doctor Humphrey?" Barbara smiled. "I had to kick Doctor Sandler out of here thirty minutes ago."

• • •

Leaving 2 East, I drove out into rural Maryland and mused about my new home, a cottage at Kirkhill Farm. For the evening hours and weekends, 2 East required more than a place to sleep, receive mail, and prepare meals. I needed to be outdoors, far away from the city.

Before my year in Germany, Frank, a fellow graduate student from the University of Chicago, invited me to share a cottage in rural Maryland when I returned for my two years at NIH. The cottage was part of an estate named Kirkhill, a half hour from work. Frank, a pediatrician and biochemist, was also a research associate and had finished his first year at NIH. He had been my graduate-school roommate for three years.

The dirt driveway led to the top of a ridge and past a stately white mansion. Fifty yards beyond was a small redbrick cottage with a slate roof. The front door and windows were framed in white, like a Currier & Ives print.

The white front door opened directly into a living room. A small sofa faced a fireplace on the far wall. To the left, a bedroom: two single beds and two very small closets. To the right, an opening to a kitchen: a sink, gas stove, refrigerator, pantry, narrow two-chair table, and kerosene heater. There was indoor plumbing, electricity, running water, and charm. As Frank said in a letter to me, "It's like a semimodern cabin by Walden Pond."

Obviously, Frank had been out scavenging antique stores. The furniture had a comfortable look. There were runners, throw rugs, a brass tray for mail, a couple of old primitive paintings, a kerosene lamp, and a few painted pots lending a bit of color. The wet nose of Shonto, Frank's lab, brushed my hand. Her chore of greeting me done, she flopped into a wicker basket.

Frank was in the kitchen reading a medical journal. "How was your first day?"

I shrugged. "Well. It's over."

"That bad?"

"I don't know. Do you mind if I give Domino an extra carrot?"

"No, of course not. He'll be your friend for life."

Out of the pasture, a black-and-white pony thundered up to the fence. Domino was a gelding—fat, sassy, and approximately thirteen hands at the withers. He had a thick mane and a disorganized forelock. His very mobile upper lip was eager for anything he could get to add to his obesity. He liked his carrot. While not a beauty, Domino was instantly likable.

Standing at the fence, I finally had time to reflect. It had been a long day, full of little things that made it unique. The Clinical Center was an attractive building on a nicely landscaped campus, 2 East was clean and well equipped, and all the rooms were private and well furnished. I wasn't dumped on the floor; the head nurse, Dee, led me down to the playroom, and a young nurse, Morgan, introduced me to my patients. I looked forward to working with Rick and Jerry. The mothers had made me feel welcome, and I really liked my three little patients.

There was a lot of studying ahead of me. I needed to read about leukemia and chemotherapy. More important, Rick was willing to show me the finer points of pediatric oncology, and I was looking forward to working with him.

Billy allowed me to hold his teddy bear. I was moved by the event at the time, and now at the fence, I figured out why: this was more than sharing; it was a statement of trust.

Domino nudged me with his muzzle, reality of the present returned, and I went in to bed.

● ● ●

My sleep had not been disturbed by fear of what awaited me on 2 East, but I awoke at six in the morning concerned about POMP. I read and started to memorize the pharmacology section of the protocol. During the drive into NIH, I repeated from memory the facts about the drugs of POMP. But chemotherapy wasn't going to be the issue of the morning.

The big problem on Wednesday, my second day on 2 East, began at a quarter to eight when a nurse met me in the hall. "You have a new patient, Doctor Humphrey. We didn't meet yesterday; my name is Brigid. I'm sorry for this interruption."

When I asked Brigid what room the patient was in, she ignored the question and continued, "It's a newborn, not yet two days old. It's a complicated case: a critically ill baby. Dee discussed the infant earlier this morning with our senior staff pediatrician. I'll tell her you're here."

The first thought through my mind was, admitted to 2 East on the first day of his life? A baby on 2 East. My shoulders drooped; I felt weak. I'd forgotten all I had learned about pediatrics as a third-year medical student. At that time, I had examined healthy newborns, but here was a sick baby, "a complicated case," and I was the doctor.

"Good morning, Doctor Humphrey," Dee said, meeting me in the hall. She paused, looked at me, and continued. "Let's go down to my office; I could use a cup of coffee."

Sitting down was a good idea.

Dee summarized a course of tragic events. "The mother is a healthy twenty-three-year-old; this was her first pregnancy. Baby Boy Williams was born at seven fifteen in the evening yesterday at Georgetown University Hospital, term, six pounds, ten ounces. The baby had tan to dark-colored cutaneous lesions, an enlarged liver and spleen, an abnormally high white count of fifty-six thousand, and a low platelet count of twenty thousand. The peripheral blood contained immature white blood cells. The baby was transferred to us by ambulance and arrived at nine oh five."

My chair squeaked as I shifted my weight.

"Doctor Karon worked up the infant, wrote orders last night, and has already seen the baby this morning. The mother is still in the hospital. Her ob-gyn wants her under observation and to keep her sedated. Doctor Karon said this is the youngest case he's ever seen. It's called infantile leukemia and is rapidly fatal. He explained that the kidneys were not functioning because of—let me find it in my notes—the accumulation of uric-acid crystals in the tubules. That's called uric-acid nephropathy." Dee looked up.

If you are trained in internal medicine, elevated uric acid suggests gout. I decided not to bother her with this information.

Together, we walked down to room 3, where the baby lay in an incubator. While nothing came to me, I washed my hands and then put them through the ports on my side of the incubator, noting an IV placed in the right leg. The baby was flaccid; his only reaction to my touch was turning his eyes toward me. Again, I had that sinking feeling.

There must have been twenty skin lesions, heart and respiratory rates were fast, and the liver and spleen were easy to palpate below the rib cage.

Instead of swearing or venting in some other way, I closed my eyes, took a deep breath, and sighed.

"Doctor Karon asked me to call after you'd seen the baby," Dee volunteered.

She had done an excellent job of presenting this case and its problems to me. "Is it Myron Karon?"

"Yes. Do you know him?"

"We were graduate students together at the University of Chicago."

My old acquaintance ambled into the room. He was short and still overweight, with dark curly hair and thick glasses, but had retained a relaxed manner I remembered well.

"Hi, Ben. I saw your name on this year's list of clinical associates. Welcome."

I started to laugh, that laugh of insecurity that can easily turn into tears.

"Yeah, I know," he continued. "You're not going to manage another baby with leukemia for the rest of your year on 2 East. This is the youngest one I've ever seen. This presentation is typical. These lesions on the skin are called leukemia cutis. The problem, the baby's problem, my problem, is that the kidneys are shut down."

"What are you going to do next?"

"I'm doing what I can. The baby is not putting out any urine. The electrolyte imbalance and renal failure are getting worse. I'll go see the mother when the baby dies. It'll probably be this morning."

Myron put both arms on top of the incubator, looked down at the baby, and straightened up. "How was your postdoc year in Germany? It was in biochemistry, wasn't it?"

"Well, it didn't prepare me for this."

"No," he said in a reflective voice. "Nothing prepares anyone for 2 East. Two years of residency in pediatrics, two years of a fellowship in pediatric oncology, and now here I am at NCI on the Leukemia Service, and I still don't feel prepared. So often it seems there's so little that we can do."

The words rolled easily off Myron's lips: "So little we can do."

This is not why I went to med school, I thought. Not to preside over death at the beginning of life.

• • •

All morning long, I was drawn to Baby Boy Williams's room. In between making rounds on John Graham, Sarah Thompkins, and Billy Sullivan, I'd look in on this almost-dead newborn. Rick and Jerry went with me to see this very rare case. These were quiet visits.

The most Brigid would say was, "There's no change."

At half past ten, while I was writing a note on Billy Sullivan's chart, Brigid came into the nurses' station. "Excuse me, Doctor Humphrey."

I turned, looked at her, and didn't have to ask. We walked to Baby Boy William's room. What had been flaccid was now lifeless. "I'll call Myron—er, Doctor Karon," I said, and Brigid removed the IV.

Myron again listened to the chest. He put his arms on top of the incubator, looked at the body of his patient, and, after a pause, said, "I'll go down to Georgetown and see Mrs. Williams."

On my bench across the street from the Clinical Center, I pondered. How could one make any sense of this infant's short life? Myron's task of telling Mrs. Williams about her son's death started to wear on my psyche. The child she had never held. For all I knew, the little boy didn't have a first name.

I got up and went for a walk.

• • •

It had to be a short walk, because I was concerned about John Graham. Bowel obstruction is a serious problem in adult medicine; I assumed the same was true in pediatrics. As I entered the room, I noted that John was sitting up, occupied with a cup of ice chips his mother held. I didn't have to ask if he was better; it was written all over their faces.

Mrs. Graham told me, "It all just started. He asked to be moved. Then he said he was hungry. Morgan clamped the suction tube and said he could have ice chips."

A broad smile on his face, John pulled the top sheet down and opened his hospital gown. It was as if he was proud of his tummy.

"John, first I'm going listen to your tummy. Will you point to where you want me to start?"

He pointed to his belly button.

"Ah, good spot. Wow! Do you know what I hear? I hear ice chips running around in your tummy. That's good! That's great!" In a growling voice, I added, "Your tummy is saying, 'When are we going to eat something?'"

That brought a big smile. The rest of the physical exam and deep palpation of the abdomen was unremarkable.

"We'll remove that tube from his nose and start him off on clear liquids, Mrs. Graham. Juices, broths, and even Jell-O. John, what's your favorite flavor of Jell-O?" I asked.

"Cherry."

I returned to examine John's abdomen again at half past twelve. "That's a good-lookin' square of Jell-O, John. Does it taste good?"

John held up his spoon and gave me an ear-to-ear smile.

An order for Jell-O in John's chart: what a simple but rewarding thing to do.

• • •

I wasn't hungry, so I continued my rounds during lunch hour with Billy Sullivan. He was sitting on his mother's lap. One hand was still taped onto an IV board, the other busy with a spoon and plate of scrambled eggs. There were bits of egg on Billy's shirt and shorts, his mother's blouse, and the chair they shared.

She noted my amusement about the eggs, shrugged, and smiled. "They put the IV in his right hand. He's very right-handed, but he doesn't like to be fed by anyone."

I noted that his teddy bear was still crusted with dried blood. "Looks like Bear needs a platelet transfusion."

"Oh," she said, "when we're home, I'll wash Bear by hand or in the machine and put him in the dryer after Billy's gone to bed. Bear's getting used to being scrubbed and tubed."

How could having leukemia become routine? "Does Billy mind having to come to the Clinical Center? How do you feel about all this?"

"Oh, you just adapt," she said, picking a freshly dropped glob of egg off her blouse and putting it back onto Billy's plate. Billy scooped up the egg and this time got it into his mouth. "Actually, Billy adapted faster than I did. I had a lot of support from other mothers here on 2 East. The nurses are good, and the doctors are helpful, but nothing beats a mom who knows chemo."

Writing my discharge orders on Billy's chart was a pleasure. Billy and his mom would be back on 2 East in ten days for his next course of POMP, and I'd be glad to see them. What a pair, I thought, a mother who could adapt and her son who just kept on going. For the future, keep Mrs. Sullivan in mind. If you have trouble with a new mother—call Billy's mom.

• • •

"Doctor Karon will explain patient management at three o'clock," Dee told us.

As we rode up to the twelfth floor, Rick said, "2 East's different. Not at all like Minneapolis or Seattle."

"Yeah, you can say that again," Jerry said. "I thought it was just me, being an internist. Oh well. Let's hope this guy Karon has something important to say. I don't need to be told NIH is a great institute; we've been carefully chosen and the rest of that kind of crap."

It *is* a strange place, I thought. A two-year-old shared his bear with me, a mother made me feel welcome, a head nurse opened a door for me, nurses took turns with a dying baby boy, and there was a pediatrician who helped internists. Most unusual of all, 2 East was a place where two internists wanted help.

We entered a small classroom off the adult leukemia nursing unit on 12 East. The two associates from the adult floor were already there, as was Myron.

"I'm Myron Karon. Welcome. We're not going to overload you with information this morning—just give you enough to keep you out of trouble."

Jerry breathed an audible sigh of relief.

"Most of your patients will have acute leukemia; a few will have a lymphoma. Only untreated patients are entered into our research program. All patients will be on the POMP protocol. Patients returning for monthly therapy are admitted Sunday night or early on Monday morning for their five-day course. This way, they can be discharged Friday afternoon. Oh, by the way, the nurses have standing orders for diet, vital signs, activity, and all that routine stuff. That means, on Sunday evening, you don't have to come in to write orders. You can do your admitting note Monday morning. The clinical associates can rotate call; for example, for you guys of 2 East, it's every third week, and it's every other week for you two on 12 East. The senior staff is always on call, and we encourage you to phone anytime there's a problem. Day or night. Tom Frei will supervise 12 East, and Jay Freireich 2 East."

Myron looked around. There were no questions.

"NCI organizes a monthly seminar on various cancer topics. You'll have a lecture on the pharmacology of cancer-chemotherapeutic agents in August from Tom Frei." Myron took a deep breath, sighed, and continued. "Jay Freireich monitors the POMP protocol. Jay will give this month's seminar on POMP next Tuesday morning at ten o'clock here. Be sure to attend."

Rick asked, "What about patients who fail POMP therapy or relapse?"

"They're eligible for an experimental drug called daunomycin," Myron said. "The protocol is available on each nurses' station."

Myron closed the orientation session with an unusual statement. "I know that in many university residency programs the house staff addresses the senior faculty as 'Doctor' or even 'Professor.' We encourage you to call us by our first name or nickname. We are, after all, all in the same boat."

That last comment was fatalistic and not like Myron, I thought. "All in the same boat," I repeated to myself. After a couple of weeks, Jerry, Rick, and I would realize that *all* was the key word. *All* meant patients, moms, nurses, clinical associates, and senior staff. *We couldn't cure 'em* was the unspoken fatalistic part. As time passed, I realized *all* also meant everybody "in the boat" bailing water together. *All* also meant acute lymphocytic leukemia.

• • •

At 3:50 p.m., Jerry's desk phone rang. "Yes, this is Doctor Sandler." With a jerk, he sat up straight. "Yes, sir. Where is your office, sir? Right away, sir. " He was out the door before we could ask if he needed any help.

Ten minutes later, Jerry returned, sat down at his desk with a plunk, and let go with a long sigh. "Ben, Rick, there's something you guys need to know. I just got chewed out for doing a tracheotomy on a patient on 12 East. My butt feels like an overworked piece of bubble gum."

"12 East? The adult leukemia ward?" Rick asked.

"Yeah, yesterday during the lunch hour. The two guys from 12 East were gone, and I was the only clinical associate they could find. An adult with a lymphoma of the neck had acute respiratory distress, so I went up and did a trach on him," Jerry said.

"Gosh, Jerry, sounds reasonable to me," Rick replied.

"Yeah. In a hospital like Bellevue, lots of patients with facial trauma, for example, needed an emergency tracheotomy, and one couldn't wait around for a surgeon to show up."

Jerry had been trained to intervene, and his rapid response to airway obstruction had probably saved a number of lives at Bellevue, I thought.

"Who chewed you out and why?" Rick asked.

"Our attending for this next year, Doctor Freireich," Jerry replied. "His response to my telling him about doing trachs at Bellevue was swift, direct, and left no room for further discussion. I was told that the Clinical Center here at NIH wasn't a public hospital; there were staff who knew what they were doing for procedures like tracheotomies. Freireich further asked if I knew the relationship between surgical hemorrhage and the platelet count, how many units of platelets I would give to an adult, and other questions I couldn't answer."

"Our attending for the next year?" I said.

He nodded. "It was all over in about three minutes, and Freireich wants the message passed on to you two. Don't do trachs. Call a surgeon."

Rick and I supported Jerry's action. How was he supposed to know? Myron hadn't said anything about procedures during his talk.

"Jerry," I said, "as you're missing half of your backside, do you need a platelet transfusion?"

Jerry laughed. "Well, next week before rounds, we could start IVs on each other and have all three of us typed and cross matched for a unit of blood. You know, just in case."

We all laughed.

The bigger question was, who was this Freireich?

• • •

At 4:05 p.m., Dee met me in the hall. "Sarah Thompkins just spiked a fever."

"Please get the bottles for a blood culture," I tried to say with my best professional persona. I had been trained to respond to problems in an objective manner, but 2 East made me feel like an amateur.

"Everything is ready in the treatment room, Doctor Humphrey," Dee said. "You'd better draw the blood for the cultures in there. Sarah is likely to have a screaming fit."

"I'll talk to the mother first and try to explain things to Sarah."

"Thanks. Morgan's already in the room. I'll help hold Sarah down. She's very strong."

Sarah lay quietly while Morgan wiped her face with a wet washcloth. Mrs. Thompkins was sitting beside her daughter, head bowed and fingertips pressed together.

In simple terms, I explained chemotherapy induced neutropenia or a low white-blood-cell count, fever, and the risk of an infection in the bloodstream.

Mrs. Thompkins listened quietly, nodding her head during my explanation. "I know. All the mothers here know about sepsis."

I had called it "an infection in the blood," but she knew the medical term, *sepsis*.

"Sarah, honey, I know I said yesterday that you'd be going home on Friday. I'm sorry, but you can't go home tomorrow."

"No! No!" she screamed. Tears rolling down her flushed cheeks, and she swung her arms widely and kicked the mattress with her heels. Sarah could not be consoled even by her mother; her screaming only abated as she exhausted herself. Dee entered the room and helped carry Sarah.

"You may come along if you wish, Mrs. Thompkins," I said.

In the center of the treatment room, under surgical lights, was a full-size operating table. Sarah was placed on her back, one restraining strap across her thighs and a second across her chest. Despite these restraints, she could still wiggle. Dee lay diagonally across the lower portion of her body and extended her hands to hold and control Sarah's left arm, which still had a working IV. Mrs. Thompkins held her daughter's head and talked in a low, quiet voice. Morgan gave me my gloves, opened a sterile IV tray, and poured povidone iodine into one cup and alcohol into a second cup. She then positioned herself to hold Sarah's right arm. I went through the vein-finding ritual, cleansing her skin, and got blood on the first stick. Dee helped Mrs. Thompkins carry a sobbing Sarah back to her room.

"That was very well done, Doctor Humphrey," Morgan said diplomatically. "Mrs. Thompkins was very helpful. Some mothers panic. Dee says that, in general, we don't encourage mothers to be present in the treatment room."

I was emotionally drained and, without thinking, said firmly, "Sarah is—Mrs. Thompkins's daughter!"

"Of course. I'm glad things went so well." Morgan collected the blood sample and left the room.

For a few minutes, I sat on a stainless-steel stool thinking about my first traumatic procedure on one of my little patients. I knew the feeling of depletion that results from maximal effort. I had run some of the most challenging rapids on the Colorado River, but that was physical exhaustion associated with exhilaration. Now I felt only emptiness. Then I thought, what the hell's wrong with you, Humphrey? You're never short with people.

In the nurses' station, Morgan was charting. "Morgan, the policy of not allowing mothers in the treatment room is right. I'll follow that rule in the future. Thanks for telling me. I'm sorry I was short with you."

"Ah—it's not my rule, Doctor Humphrey. There are, of course, exceptions." Morgan dropped her pen, unprepared for my apology.

Dee interrupted. "Doctor Humphrey, we have a protocol for sepsis. I made a copy for you and thought you might want to read it before you wrote antibiotic orders on Sarah."

"Thank you. Thanks a lot." I took it and Sarah's chart and retreated to the doctors' office. The protocol contained tables, graphs, names of pathological bacteria and their sensitivity to various antibiotics, practical information, and specific recommendations.

I must remember: pediatric patients scream and cry; don't take your frustration out on a nurse, and never tell patients that you'll discharge them tomorrow, or at the end of the week, or that they can go home if everything is all right.

I had performed one procedure, technically well done but not truly well. I wasn't proud of my behavior and wondered how I was going to get through the year.

After a polite knock on the door, Morgan entered the office. "I thought you might like a cup of coffee, Doctor Humphrey."

• • •

I poked around 2 East until 6:10. I went to the cafeteria for dinner and was back by 6:40 p.m.

As I walked into the nurses' station, Barbara handed me Sarah's chart open to the vital signs page. In a very quiet voice, she said, "Sarah's going to be all right, Doctor Humphrey."

Barbara didn't have to tell me to go home. It had been a long day.

• • •

Friday, July 3, was a holiday, but we hardly noticed. The patients were still on the floor receiving their last day of POMP. The nurses were taking care of them, and the three of us had agreed to come in Friday morning to discharge those patients who had finished their five-day course and to evaluate our patients that had to stay in the hospital over the weekend. The nation was celebrating Independence Day but not the children of 2 East.

Rick, Jerry, and I met at noon.

"I'll take call," Rick said.

"Thanks, I'd appreciate that."

"Well, Ben, you've had a death—the baby. Some time off might be good," Rick said.

"I've seen a lot of patients die in Bellevue, but I think it's going to be different here."

Silence fell.

Finally Jerry said, "Rick, all my patients have been discharged."

"I have Sarah Thompkins, fever and low white count. Her blood cultures of Thursday afternoon are still sterile. I also have John Graham, abdominal lymphoma. His bowel obstruction has responded to radiation therapy. We're advancing his diet."

"OK. Got it," Rick said.

"By the way, Sarah doesn't like clinical associates."

"Well, some are like that. Toddlers all the way through adolescents."

"But they can be damned affectionate," Jerry said. "I discharged a four-year-old girl this morning, Susan. On the way out, she broke away from her mother, ran back, took my hand, squeezed it, looked up, giggled, and then ran back to her mother."

"I have only one patient in the hospital. I'm concerned about her condition. Jennifer Johnson, seven, neutropenic, febrile, and she has a small ulcer on her lower lip," Rick said.

"Well, she's in good hands," Jerry said.

Our clinical reports and anecdotes over, the three of us exchanged some personal information.

"I've rented an apartment in Georgetown," Jerry said. "Short walk for coffee and a croissant for breakfast but a longer walk for bars and restaurants in the evening."

"My wife, Jody, and I rent a small house in Chevy Chase. Our first home. No more apartments for us," Rick said.

"I've a cottage out in rural Maryland near Darnestown. It's actually a guest house on an estate complete with barn and a fenced-in fourteen-acre pasture. I'm gonna buy and train a young Thoroughbred."

"You're going to buy a horse? Spend time with a horse? DC is full of unattached women," Jerry exclaimed.

"I'll buy a mare, Jerry."

Rick smiled, shaking his head as if to say, "Am I going to have to work with these two clowns for a year?"

Jerry and I came to love this gesture.

We were in no hurry. We sat together and enjoyed each other's company. No longer three physicians from different parts of the country and different medical schools, we were just three guys thrown together on a leukemia ward. Time together was like R&R.

• • •

Much of Montgomery County lay outside of time and dozed in a midafternoon of the twentieth century. In 1964, that meant the small crossroad towns, like Darnsetown, Poolsville, Quince Orchard, and Germantown, were joined by two-lane roads. There were few stop signs on the roads or in the towns, and they weren't necessary as local traffic moved slowly. Sprinkled throughout the county were white steepled churches waiting for Sunday. The denizens had deep roots in the rich soil. Their families had lived in Montgomery for generations before the war, and by that they meant the War between the States.

I arrived back at Kirkhill to meet Mindy, Frank's riding instructor, who drove over from Poolesville. She jumped out of a one-ton red four-wheel-drive Ford pickup with a long bed. A serious horse trailer–pulling vehicle. An attractive young woman of average height, an expressive face with large eyes, her blond hair in a ponytail, Mindy wore English riding attire. Her britches revealed strong legs. I was willing to bet she could do three-gaited, five-gaited, jump or cut cattle. I would wager there wasn't a horse in the county she couldn't handle.

"Hi. Frank. This must be your friend Ben. Let's get out of the sun," Mindy said. "I want to know about Ben's experiences with horses so I can fix you boys up with a couple of Thoroughbreds. Have you ever owned a horse, Ben?"

"Never have. During high school, I worked at a rich kids' camp in the Rhinelander area of northern Wisconsin where I cared for twelve school horses. All mares, except the riding master's personal stallion. Forking manure, grooming, and saddling the horses for morning and afternoon riding classes was good exercise."

"Well, that's a damned good start."

"The riding master taught me some of the finer points of three-gaited riding such as collecting your mount, knowing what lead the horse was in, changing leads, and so on."

"OK. You can care for 'em and ride 'em. You ever been thrown?"

"Not yet."

"Then you've got a lot to learn," she said and tossed me a smile. "Anything else?"

"Two years ago, my last year in Chicago, I took lessons and rode tennessee walkers. Frank told me this is Thoroughbred country. I have no wish to look for a walker."

"Good! Walkers aren't common in the state. Besides, Thoroughbreds are cheap and plentiful."

"Cheap? Why's that?"

"There's a lot of claiming races here. My husband's a cop. We train, race, and breed Thoroughbreds. It's a hobby, but we do make a little money at it. My family's been raising Thoroughbreds for a long time. At any rate, if a horse isn't fast enough, they're sold to people like you and Frank or slaughtered for meat. We'll get a horse that only knows how to break out of a starting gate. Your job will be to teach 'em to walk, trot, and canter. Well, you boys have a good day; I've got to go."

Frank and I watched her climb into the cab and drive off.

"She's a great human being, Doctor Thorp. I can see why you like her. After four years of being 'Doctor' or 'Herr Doctor,' I enjoy being called a 'boy.'"

• • •

Saturday morning. Space was limited in the cabin. Frank was tidy, and I was more disorganized, so I needed to organize my stuff. Stashed in a box in one corner of the bedroom were books from graduate school and my year in Germany. Like a dog at the door, they had waited for my return; now was time for our reunion.

I arranged my books in four piles. Three very special paperbacks constituted a small stack. I would select one of these three to accompany me when I went camping, skiing, backpacking, or running the Colorado River: Louis Untermeyer's *A Concise Treasury of Great Poems*,

Huston Smith's *The Religions of Man,* and Blakney's translation of the *Tao Te Ching.*

Pile two: a German collection. Friends in Mainz had given me several books including Norton's English translation of Rainer Maria Rilke poems. I smiled as I leafed through a paperback of folk songs.

Next were two novels by Remarque. *All Quiet on the Western Front* in English haunted me. I especially related to Paul Brennen, a young man who as a child collected butterflies. While in Germany, I thought reading another novel, *Drie Kamaraden,* by Remarque, in German would be a good exercise.

The last to be shelved were used books collected from stores around the University of Chicago—each one a diamond found in a heap of irrelevant tomes.

Hanging up my clothes didn't take any time at all as I had very few items.

Finally I opened a case with a long neck. My five-string Kay banjo, the capo attached, welcomed me back to memories of evenings with friends and songfests on the ski bus to Colorado. Before closing the case, I found a *Peanuts* cartoon I had clipped. After the birth of Charlie Brown's sister, Sally, Snoopy is lying on top of his doghouse and thinks, "Every baby should be issued a banjo at birth."

• • •

Sunday evening. Time to reflect on the past six days and to fear tomorrow. I had completed the first week; I hadn't killed anyone or missed anything to the best of my knowledge. I only hoped I could say the same at the end of the next week. It looked like my life was going to unfold one week at a time.

Frank had left the farm in the late afternoon to go into Bethesda, where he probably had a date or wanted to complete work in his lab. He didn't tell me what he was going to do or when he'd be back. That was typical of our relationship. We didn't keep track of each other.

The weekend, all too short, had been a good break, almost good enough to forget 2 East. But not quite. The excitement about getting my first horse had abated.

A sheet of lightweight blue paper lay before me on the kitchen table. I had promised to write Kristina. I'd dated her during my last six months in Mainz. The aerogram was blank, but my mind was full of images of forests above the Rhine River.

July 5, 1964

Dear Kristina:

It's been over three weeks since our last walk in the Neiderwald. I remember the picnic lunch we bought in Ruhdesheim and looking down on the Rhine during our hike. I can now go outside of my cabin in rural Maryland and look down at a large fenced-in meadow. The view is nice but not as romantic as the Rhine River Valley.

I call this a cabin because it is small: one bedroom, a living room with a fireplace, a small kitchen, and a bathroom. It is a thirty-minute drive from my work at the National Institutes of Health.

I've made arrangements to buy a horse, which will be delivered next weekend. I'll write you about that in a week or two.

Sorry for such a short note. It's late, and I'm tired. I've written in English. We both know that your English is vastly superior to my German.

Love,
Ben

I looked at the letter. An aerogram covered in ink from a ballpoint pen. There were facts but not a word of truth about the life I was living. I folded it carefully along the dotted lines and went to bed.

Second Week

Monday morning's trip into NIH was a drive into uncertainty. Had anybody been admitted for terminal care? Any nosebleeds? Any admission for a sudden fever that might represent the threat of fatal sepsis? God only knew what might happen. I mulled over the significance of the first full week on 2 East. Rick would tell me about John Graham's diet and Sarah Thompkins's risk of bacterial sepsis. We'd find out how Jennifer Johnson was doing.

"Good morning, Rick. Hi, Jerry. How was call, Rick?"

"Your two kids are both doing fine, Ben. Sarah has been afebrile, and her blood cultures still show no growth. You can probably stop the IV antibiotics today. John has been eating up a storm—gained a kilo since Friday."

"Thanks." I paused, looking into Rick's face. "What's wrong, Rick?"

"I've got a problem. A real big problem." He reviewed the progress of Jennifer's mouth lesion and then discussed toxicity. "Methotrexate does that. In Minnesota, any sign of mucositis, and we stopped therapy, especially methotrexate. When I wrote the order to hold Jennifer's POMP on Friday, Dee said I had better talk to Karon. When I did, Myron told me that the protocol stated that therapy was not to be stopped, and that was the way Freireich wanted it. In my two-year fellowship in oncology, I've never seen anything like this. Come on, guys, I'd better show you."

Jennifer lay on her back, motionless, eyes closed. Her lips were swollen, cracked, and coated with dried blood, the tissue around the mouth red and swollen, especially on the right side. The swelling extended to the lower face and down into her neck. We stared at her, silent with disbelief.

Out in the hall, Rick explained, "You don't have to look for the first evidence of methotrexate-induced mouth ulcers. The kids will tell you about 'em, and Jennifer initially had one small superficial ulcer on her right lower lip on Thursday. She hasn't eaten since. It's progressed every day. Now she has staph growing in her blood. She's on antibiotics, IV fluids, platelet transfusion to control bleeding, IV albumin for caloric support, and morphine." Shaking his head, he said, "I didn't know it could be this bad."

Jerry and I watched Rick trudge down the hall. It wasn't just his problem.

• • •

Dee asked to see all three of us about the admitting routine for Monday mornings. She did not start the meeting with a smile. She had seen us standing outside of Jennifer's room with Rick and knew if there had been pleasures from the weekend, these had evaporated.

"Doctor Lottsfeldt, you have one admission today: Jasper Thomas. His mother is very quiet. Doctor Sandler, you have two admissions, both outgoing kids. Doctor Humphrey, Doctor Freireich called this morning. He wants John Graham started on POMP. You have one admission, Sally Carter. She's three and a half and a real chatterbox."

Dee ended with a short overview. On a "good Monday," there might be only one or two admissions for each physician. On a "bad Monday," there could be as many as three or more. To help organize all of this, Dee explained the purpose of "the Board," a large white board hanging in the nurses' station. Using black felt-tip markers, the nurses wrote the name of the patient, the patient's age and sex, the room number, and an abbreviation for what procedures were scheduled: BM, bone-marrow aspiration; LP, lumbar puncture; IV, intravenous-needle placement for infusion of fluids, chemotherapy, or blood products. There were three lists, one for each clinical associate. The Board could easily be read from the hall, so the physicians didn't have to ask what was required for the morning. On Tuesday or thereafter, if an extra procedure was required, that was written in red. After these extra procedures were done, the red ink was erased.

The Board could also be read by the older patients. The little ones, some with tears in their eyes, would ask, "Is my name on the Board in red?"

• • •

Rick, I've busted into the bone-marrow cavity of adults, you know; we aspirated the marrow out of the sternum. What do you do with a five-year-old?" Jerry asked.

"Let's go down to the treatment room. I'll tell you about marrow aspirates, and then you guys can watch me do one," Rick said.

"My boss in Minnesota stressed, 'Inform the mother of a newly diagnosed case of what's going to happen because it's going to happen every month.' Comment on how painful a bone-marrow procedure is. The skin can be deadened with Xylocaine, but even that hurts. Tell the mom that the membrane over the surface of the bone is very sensitive, that when this membrane, the periosteum, is torn or punctured, there is intense pain, like when a bone breaks. There is also a lot of pain when the marrow is sucked out of the cavity. It's not just another needlestick."

Rick went on to explain the position: patient on his or her tummy, a nurse holding the shoulders. If necessary, a second nurse might have to immobilize the hips by holding the upper thighs. The marrow is drawn out of the posterior crest of the hip.

Brigid carried a whimpering five-year-old boy into the treatment room.

Rick's little patient screamed on being held, screamed when the Xylocaine was injected, screamed when the periosteum was infiltrated, screamed when the skin was penetrated with the aspiration needle, screamed when the needle was drilled through the bone, and screamed when the marrow was aspirated. This was followed by uncontrollable sobbing, soft crying, and gasping for breath.

I wanted to sit down. Yes, moms needed to know why this was necessary. I now realized that hurting a five-year-old or any patient would also be traumatic for me, but a different kind of trauma.

I was going to spend a year breaking little bones.

• • •

"Hi, Doctor H.," Morgan said in a peppy voice. A smile on her round face was complemented by her bright-brown eyes beneath her auburn bangs. "You're in for a treat. That's Sally Carter and her mom that Brigid is taking down to her room."

Short of stature, Mrs. Carter was wearing cork-wedged shoes, and her blond hair was up in a beehive. Her light-blue sleeveless top matched her pedal pushers. Her bald daughter, Sally, carried a doll that was almost half as tall as she was. The doll had tannish hair pulled into a bun on the top of its head and wore a loose-fitting leopard-patterned gown.

By the time I got into the room, Sally was sitting on her mother's lap, clutching her doll. "Hi, Sally, I'm Doctor Humphrey."

No response. After saying good morning to Mrs. Carter, I asked why Sally was so quiet.

"Give her about half an hour, and you'll be blessed with an outpouring of words, stories, and even a few questions." Mrs. Carter provided me with a good review of the previous courses of POMP.

"What's the name of your doll, Sally?" I asked.

Sally looked at me with an incredulous frown, glanced at her mom, and then said, "Pebbles."

"That's a cute name. Unusual too," I said.

Sally's frown softened, but she held her head in an angle of uncertainty. If you're three years old and your doctor doesn't know who Pebbles is, you probably think you've got a dumb doctor. Mrs. Carter explained that Pebbles was from *The Flintstones*.

Mrs. Carter helped me with the physical examination, reassuring Sally that everything was all right. I was about to leave when the thirty-minute grace period ended.

"I have a friend. Her name's Betsy."

I sat down to listen.

"Her doll's a Raggedy Ann. Do you know Raggedy Ann?"

I started to say I knew the Raggedy Ann doll when Sally continued.

"They have red hair. I don't like red hair."

With a casual touch of Sally's shoulder, a signal that was understood by both mother and daughter, Sally stopped talking, and Mrs. Carter explained, "It's Monday, Sally, and Doctor Humphrey has a lot of things to do."

What a team! I went over to my verbose little patient and touched the other shoulder. "In a day or two, I want to hear all about Betsy, and maybe you can tell me about *The Flintstones*."

Out in the hall, I thought, Sally's more than a chatterbox; she's charming. Among the things you have to do, Humphrey, is go to a children's bookstore and leaf through a children's book on *The Flintstones*. That might be more fun than reading the next issue of *Cancer Research*.

• • •

If you misspell a word on the chart, nobody will die. If you miscalculate the dose of a medicine, someone could.

Since we had started our clinical exposure to pediatric oncology midweek, the POMP orders had been written by last year's clinical associates. Jerry and I had been spared one week of having to divine the actual doses of the drugs.

Two things bothered me. First of all, I had never prescribed methotrexate, 6-mercaptopurine, or vincristine for any patient. This was the lesser of my two problems. Thank God, the POMP protocol had a pharmacology section that outlined in great detail the formulation, mechanism of action, toxicity, and therapeutic experience of each drug. Now, I was about to put pen to paper on an order sheet.

Toxicity: an image of Jennifer's swollen neck and bleeding lips appeared before me.

My bigger problem was the method to calculate the dose of each drug. It was not based on age or weight but the body surface area. I had never used the BSA. The doses of many drugs in adult medicine are the same for a twenty-year-old and a sixty-year-old, someone thin and someone fat. In contrast, the BSA is calculated from the patient's height in centimeters and weight in kilograms and reported in meters squared.

OK, I had a safety net with Sally's orders. I calculated her BSA and the doses for POMP and then compared my conclusion with those written the previous month. I got the BSA and doses of all four drugs right.

John Graham was a different story. He had not previously received POMP. I was on my own. Jennifer's swollen face remained in my mind. I went through the same procedure and wrote the orders. At eleven years of age, John was taller and weighed more than Sally, but I had no way of knowing if his BSA was correct and his doses appropriate. I began to think of my ballpoint pen as a smoking gun.

In the nurses' station, I handed the orders to a very young nurse named Sharon. "Please check these orders before you send them to the pharmacy. If I have made a mistake, let me know, and I'll be glad to rewrite 'em." Her eyes opened wide, and her jaw dropped. I walked back to the doctors' office where I started a list of questions for Rick.

Ten minutes later, I heard a gentle knock on the door. Dee asked if she could come in.

"These orders are fine, Doctor Humphrey. You startled Sharon; she's only been on the floor for two weeks. It's a little unusual for a physician to ask for his orders to be checked by a nurse. I explained that everybody on the floor was upset about Jennifer and you wished to do everything possible to prevent this type of toxicity."

"Dee, how long have you been reading chemotherapy orders?" I said, irritated.

"For a number of years."

"Well then, your experience exceeds mine. I do not wish to inadvertently contribute to the toxicity that's so abundant on this floor," I snapped. I was about to say I didn't give a rat's rump what some young nurse thought but caught myself.

"Doctor Humphrey, we'll help in any way we can." She was calm and experienced in dealing with clinical associates. "I'll be glad to look over your chemotherapy orders. Barbara, the short white-haired nurse, also has a lot of experience. I think it's commendable you're willing to ask us for help." She smiled and left.

What's wrong with you, Humphrey? You've been down this road before. I thought back to my first rotation on the Cardiology Service as an intern at the University of Chicago Clinics and Hospital. I considered digitalis a tricky and potentially dangerous drug, so I always asked my resident to check those orders. After two weeks, the professor of cardiology asked to see me in his office. He told me in fatherly terms he thought I was doing a good job, but I didn't have to show my orders to the resident. Part of the training in an internship was assuming responsibility, he told me, and next year, as a resident, I'd be in charge of a team. I remember thanking him and realizing, you're now an MD.

The door to Dee's small office was always open. I knocked.

"Come in, Doctor Humphrey."

"I apologize for being short with you. That's not my nature, and my attitude was inappropriate. Being at 2 East is not bringing out the best in me."

"Oh no." She pushed herself back from the pile of papers on her desk. "You weren't short in your remarks. We're all edgy about POMP. It is very toxic. To be honest, I always look over the orders. And pharmacy staff always wants to know the patient's height and weight. They recalculate the BSA and check the doses too."

"That's great," I laughed, breaking the tension. "Keep it up. I've got an idea. We'll call 2 East a dog shelter. Let's classify the patients as puppies. I'll call the Humane Society, and they'll shut the place down." I was on a roll but decided to stop. I didn't want to find myself before a firing squad for insubordination. We were both laughing. It felt good.

In the nurses' station, I found Sharon. She straightened her posture.

"Sharon, I'm sorry. I didn't know you'd only been on the floor a couple of weeks. I'm glad you gave my orders to Dee."

She relaxed, her shoulders dropping slightly. "Oh, Doctor, I just didn't know what to do with your orders. I've so much to learn. I just hope I can…Nothing in nursing school prepared me for this."

"I know."

What I didn't know this second week in July was that it was caring for the children of 2 East that was getting to me. I called them patients. I had a lot to learn.

• • •

Tuesday morning, 7:40 a.m. I opened the door to the doctors' office and saw Rick at his desk.

"How's Jennifer?"

"Worse."

"How could she be worse?"

"Yesterday, when each dose of morphine wore off, she'd open her eyes and look at her mom, and tears would roll down her cheeks. Now she's comatose—doesn't open her eyes or move."

I just nodded.

Jerry walked in. "How's Jennifer?"

• • •

How could anybody justify the toxicity of POMP?

The clinical associates from 12 East were already in the classroom. Doctor Emil J. Freireich entered at exactly ten o'clock and made a few semipolite welcoming sounds as if he were following some sort of social protocol. He was tall and blocky, neither fat nor muscular. Short slightly curly black hair topped an oval face scarred from battles with adolescent acne. He said we were to call him Jay.

Friereich started with the background on chemotherapy in leukemia. He often used the blackboard to write the statistical analysis of this or that clinical trial. During this presentation, he tended to hold his left hand at shoulder level. His fist was closed. Four drugs had been identified that could cause a clinical remission: the four drugs of POMP. Sequential use of these drugs hadn't cured anyone. Two-drug combinations caused more patients to go into remission that lasted for several months, but all patients relapsed and died. The fist remained closed. Chemotherapy during the first remission was the best chance for developing curative therapy. His other hand was open and the index finger raised. Previous four-drug trials at NCI had demonstrated improvement over two-drug combinations. The median duration of remission for one of these four-drug combinations, called VAMP (*v*incristine, *a*methoperin, 6-*m*ercaptopurine, and *p*rednisone), was nine months. Similar results were obtained with another trial called BIKE (cycles of different drugs). The hand was now open.

Freireich explained that he, Doctor Frie, and Doctor Karon had used the VAMP experience to design POMP. It wasn't a lecture. It was more like a verbal attack on leukemia. He was so intense one could not imagine falling asleep or even daydreaming. It was clear that Emil J. Freireich was dedicated to curing leukemia. That was good. What bothered me was the nature of the research. It was guided by practical experience or trial and error and not by theory. When I was a graduate student, this was often discussed as basic research versus applied research. Basic research or theoretical research was the sacred cow of science, as far as

I was concerned. Intellectually, I knew that a lot of very valuable drugs were found by stumbling around in the darkness of empirical research. Digitalis for heart failure was a good example, but I was still idealistic and very young; research, I believed, should be based on science.

Freireich's tirade had taken about thirty minutes. His eyes narrowed. He looked the five of us over to see if there were any questions.

"I'll be glad to manage the patients on my ward," one of the 12 East associates started to say.

"Doctor, you don't manage 12 East." Jay paused. "You follow the protocol. Do the bone marrows, write the orders, and keep my patients on the POMP schedule. This is not a ward in a county hospital full of the dregs of humanity dumped there by the police or a society that doesn't care what happens to them. This is not a ward for medical students to practice their juvenile therapeutic skills with little or no supervision."

A couple of chairs scratched the floor as some of us shifted our weight from one haunch to another.

We squirmed under his stare until Rick cleared his throat.

"Uh, I understand that we are to follow the protocol," he said. "We're to start the chemotherapy on schedule, but when a patient develops toxicity such as mucositis in the middle of a course of POMP, shouldn't therapy be stopped? Or at least the last doses of methotrexate? That's what we would have done in Minnesota."

"You're not in Minnesota. You're on the Leukemia Service of the National Institute of Cancer," Jay said sharply.

Jerry and I straightened up. Rick was going through hell about Jennifer and didn't deserve an attack for trying to prevent this kind of toxicity in the future.

Jerry asked, "Have you seen Jennifer?"

"I've seen worse."

"She's on morphine," I added.

"That's what morphine is for, Doctor Humphrey."

I settled back in my chair, looking down at the floor.

Finally Freireich fired his parting shot. "So, Doctor Lottsfeldt, you want to stop treatment. You want to give the leukemia cells hidden throughout her body a chance to multiply and cause a relapse. You don't get it! You're not here to prevent toxicity. You're not here to keep patients comfortable. You're here to keep patients in remission. Patients can get over toxicity. They can't get over a relapse!"

Jay looked at the five of us and left the room with its blackboard full of statistics. We stood up and went back to our patients on POMP.

Silence gives consent.

The three of us rode the elevator down to 2 East. So that is the captain, I thought.

Jerry finally broke the silence. "What a heartless schmuck!"

$$\bullet \quad \bullet \quad \bullet$$

Back on 2 East, Brigid, the quiet and calm nurse who was with me when Baby Boy Williams died, said to me, "I hope you don't mind my commenting on John's level of stress, but I hate to see a child living in such constant terror. Some kids just stop eating, others are nauseated, and some vomit a couple of times, but John vomits, trembles, and retches. He's been that way all morning."

"Mind?" I said. "Just the opposite, Brigid. I appreciate your sharing that with me."

We entered John's room. The air was rancid from vomited food. Mrs. Graham was at John's side, holding his hand. With his free hand, John clutched the yellow-stained sheet to his chest.

"I've been telling John that this vomiting is due to the drugs. Not the tumor that caused him to get sick," Mrs. Graham said. "Barbara explained that to both of us last night."

I approached the bedside. John shifted his weight toward his mother. I started to say his mother was right and reached out to touch his shoulder, but he turned away.

With a little verbal reassurance and physical help from his mother, John let me examine his abdomen. I told him, "I can't feel that tumor, and I heard those good bowel sounds." I offered John my stethoscope and asked if he would like to listen. He shook his head. I told Mrs. Graham I'd return after lunch.

Over sandwiches, I told Rick that John not trusting me was logical, but I hated to think what was going on in his head every time he vomited.

Rick suggested I try drawings. "Some kids will get it with a picture."

Later, armed with a pad and a pencil, I entered John's room and explained to Mrs. Graham what I was going to do. Brigid had asked to be present to help.

I asked what word John used for vomiting and was told *puke.* I outlined a man, drew a tube from the mouth to stomach going directly to the bottom of the abdomen. That was the healthy John. I added a black blob in the abdomen, the tumor, and then drew puke coming out of the mouth. I reminded John of the x-ray treatments and erased some of the black blob and the puke. Then I added an IV in the arm, drew in arrows from the IV to the tumor, and erased a little more of the black blob. I drew additional arrows from the IV up to the head and added puke. It was my best shot at a lecture on tumor obstruction and vomiting and chemotherapy stimulating the vomiting center in the brain. Turning to a fresh sheet of paper, I drew the figure without an IV, with no puke, standing in front of his home. I even added a shining sun.

Mrs. Graham looked at John and said, "We'll go home and tell this story to Dad."

"I'll see if I can use this approach to explain why John has to come back in a month," she said. "You know, a tiny black spot that we need to get rid of."

Out in the hall, Brigid said, "I like this idea."

"Doctor Lottsfeldt suggested it." I looked at my watch. 1:47 p.m. "Well, rounds with Doctor Freireich coming up. Thanks for your help."

• • •

Two o'clock. Our first rounds with Freireich—no time was wasted. My patients were on schedule, and so were Jerry's. Rick presented one patient for monthly POMP and then summarized the clinical data on Jennifer.

It was all over in fifteen minutes, but Jerry threw down the gauntlet. "Would you like to see Jennifer, Doctor Freireich? Mrs. Johnson is going through hell."

We followed Jay. He knew which room was Jennifer's. He sat down next to Mrs. Johnson; she gave him her hand and leaned forward. During their inaudible exchange, time was suspended. When she leaned back in her chair, Jay shook her hand. She thanked him for coming in again.

Doctor Freireich left 2 East without saying a word, leaving us to wonder if there was a human being inside this schmuck.

• • •

Tuesday afternoon dragged on. We moved in and out of the office, the nurses' station, and patient rooms. Jerry and I wondered if we should ask Rick about Jennifer. We questioned whether that would be supportive. Remembering Myron's "we are all in the same boat," we went together to see her.

The room was quiet, the air heavy with a deodorant trying unsuccessfully to mask the odor of infected flesh. Mrs. Thompkins was there, standing next to Jennifer's mom. Morgan was at the bedside changing a dressing that covered Jennifer's lower face and neck.

Rick put on gloves and lifted the dressing. It was as if there were no skin—just red swollen tissue, clotted blood, and reddish-yellow opaque fluid that oozed onto the gauze. Rick didn't have to look at either Jerry or me to ask whether we had seen enough. He replaced the dressing, took off his gloves, and went over to Jennifer's mom. Jerry and I went back to the office.

At 4:20 p.m., as I walked down the hall, Morgan and Rick rushed into Jennifer's room.

Twenty minutes later, Rick came into the office, dropped in his chair, opened a chart, and started to write.

When Jerry heard him close the chart, he asked, "Jennifer?"

Rick nodded. "I don't ever again want to see this kind of toxicity. It's not acceptable."

This coming from a man who had spent two years training in oncology and was planning to be a full-time pediatric oncologist at the University of Washington.

• • •

Wednesday morning, I went to Sally's room and sat down on the end of her bed. "Tell me about Betsy."

"She's very pretty."

"Does she have curly hair?"

"No."

"Well, I think—"

She interrupted, "One of her dolls has curly hair. Curly black hair."

I smiled and chuckled. Just nod, I thought. That'll keep Sally's monologue going. This three-year-old was sharing her life with me, telling me what was important, how she felt about things. I lacked the insight to ask myself, why can't you do that, Humphrey?

"Thank you, Doctor Humphrey, for taking time just to be with Sally," Mrs. Carter said. "You're very patient. We need that, especially after Jennifer."

"It's not a matter of being patient, Mrs. Carter. This is I something I *like* to do." I had planned on saying that, but it was true.

• • •

Jerry and I asked Rick to join us for a cup of coffee.

"Rick, the moms know about Jennifer," I said.

"And I've been asked, 'Why does the therapy have to be so toxic?'" Jerry added.

Rick shrugged. "And you two want to know how to handle this topic. So did we at Minnesota, and the protocols we used didn't begin to have the toxicity we're seeing on 2 East."

"What did you tell that mom, Jerry?" I asked.

"I sat down and listened to her. Then told her nobody liked POMP: the three of us and the nurses. Finally, I said lower doses are less toxic, but the duration of remission is shorter. You know, the data right out of Freireich's lecture."

"I'd be willing to bet toxicity even bothers Jay." Rick said in a reflective tone. "Remember how he sat and listened to Jennifer's mom."

"Being willing to listen and willing to talk may be the best we can do, but it's a little short on why," I said.

"You might try this," Rick said. "I've explained to a couple of moms the idea of the therapeutic index. An effective dose of penicillin kills germs and is basically nontoxic. An effective dose of methotrexate that kills leukemia cells is already toxic. You can increase the dose of penicillin, and you still don't get any toxicity. Penicillin is a safe drug. You can't increase the dose of methotrexate without serious life-threatening toxicity." He concluded by saying that parents don't necessarily need to know the name and therapeutic index, but they do need to know the principle. "Parents will do almost anything to treat their child's leukemia. Some find that understanding helps them cope."

• • •

During the previous year, I had not used the arcane language of medicine.

47

When I asked Rick about mothers using technical terms, he said, "Well, Ben, I can tell you what my boss in Minnesota said. He told me, '*Never* talk down to a mom, and don't hide behind jargon.'"

OK, Humphrey, I thought. You're dealing with some great mothers. Use both the medical term and the lay term.

The POMP protocol and my copy of Wintrobe's textbook *Clinical Hematology* were both necessary for me to reacquaint myself with some specific medical terms. The textbook was my first priority. First, I reviewed the pathological terms associated with leukemia. These malignant cells at diagnosis were found not only in the blood but also in almost every organ in the body. One of the most common clinical signs was abdominal distension due to enlargement of the liver, called *hepatomegaly*, and spleen, called *splenomegaly*. As the normal cells of bone marrow were crowded out by the leukemic cells, no red blood cells or erythrocytes were produced, resulting in anemia. *Granulocytopenia* was the medical term for the lack of healthy white blood cells normally produced to fight infection. No white blood cells could result in an infection from either a bacterium or a virus.

Some of the most frightening presentations were hemorrhages due to lack of production of platelets. These small packages of clot-promoting molecules controlled bleeding. Profuse nosebleeds could cause significant loss of blood. Small hemorrhages in the skin produced small punctate red dots called *petechiae*.

Cancer chemotherapy included some important new terms and concepts for me. *Induction therapy* referred to the use of drugs to eliminate leukemic cells from the bone marrow, thus causing a remission. Aspirated cells from the marrow appeared to contain normal cells. *Minimal residual disease* referred to the concept that small numbers of leukemic cells remained in the body during the remission state. *Maintenance therapy* referred to the use of drugs to suppress or try to eliminate the residual leukemic cells. The reoccurrence of leukemia in the bone marrow was called a *relapse*. The relapsed leukemic cells had acquired resistance to the antileukemic action of the drugs used during the remission maintenance therapy.

• • •

By Friday afternoon, all three of us were in a good mood. None of the remaining patients were at imminent risk of dying, and all were going to finish POMP today.

"Ah, Jerry, after Freireich's lecture, you called him a *schmuck*. I've heard the word, but I'm not sure I know how to use it," Rick said.

I laughed.

"How is it you know Yiddish, Ben?" Jerry asked.

"Well, at the University of Chicago, a third of my friends in graduate school were Jewish," I said. "Some of them had a great sense of humor, especially when using Yiddish to tell a joke. When I told my dad I was learning a little Yiddish, he laughed, saying, 'Some Jewish jokes can't be translated.'"

"Rick," Jerry said, "*schmuck* means penis, but applied to an individual like Freireich, it means SOB or prick. It can also mean someone you don't respect or like. It's very vulgar." Jerry looked at Rick.

Jerry and I exchanged a couple of our favorite schmuck jokes.

One of my favorite jokes was about a Jew who moved to Miami. "He wanted to break into society. Everything he tried failed until he bought a camel and rode it every day. But one day, his camel was stolen. He called the police who wanted a description of the animal. He knew his camel's height and the color of its coat, but he didn't know its sex. That's an important fact the police said. 'Oh I remember,' the Jew said, 'it's a male.' 'Are you sure,' the policeman asked? 'Yes,' the Jew said. 'The other day I was riding and someone yelled, look at the schmuck on that camel.'"

Jerry's was about two horny goyim. "Richard and William, walking down Main Street with Moshe, their boss. They spied an oil lamp. With a rub, out popped a genie. 'You get one wish a piece,' said the genie. Richard shouted. 'I want make love all day long to a beautiful Blonde on a yacht in Bermuda!' Poof. He disappeared. William exclaimed, 'Make mine two blondes in Hawaii!' Poof, he was gone. Moshe, the boss, looked around and calmly said. 'For my wish ... I want those schmucks back in my office right after lunch!'"

Rick nodded and flashed his special smile that Jerry and I loved. "Am I going to have to work with you two clowns for a whole year?"

Rick could teach me how to care for my little patients and communicate with their moms; Jerry would enrich my knowledge of Yiddish. I would need both to survive.

• • •

Saturday morning. Jerry had volunteered to take call, so I could be at Kirkhill. Having cared for horses, I helped Frank with the purchases of halters, leads, a lunge line and whip, saddle soap, buckets, and other necessary stuff. The Thoroughbreds were to be delivered midday.

During breakfast, Frank asked, "Did you like being a stableboy?"

"Oh yeah. I enjoyed the smell of a horse and thought forking manure was good for my muscles. Besides, shoveling shit is good training for academic medicine."

After breakfast, I witnessed a ritual played out between Frank's pony, Domino, and his black lab. Shonto liked to sit in the watering tank to cool off, but she was always alert as she looked out into the pasture.

Noting the occupant in his drinking water, Domino interrupted his grazing and charged up the hill. At the very last moment, Shonto would jump out of the tank and scoot under the lower strand of barbed wire. Her timing was perfect. Domino would nicker; Shonto would wag her tail and shake water from her coat. Domino never stayed to guard the tank. Gluttony would call him back to the pasture. Once he was grazing,

Shonto would slip back into the tank, and the show started all over. Both enjoyed the game.

Right on time, midday, Mindy's horse trader, John Simmons, rolled up the drive in a clean metallic-green pickup and matching two-horse trailer

I introduced myself. Mr. Simmons was rather short, very thin, and white haired with a narrow David Niven mustache. He was dressed in lightweight pants, and his boots were clean.

"Good afternoon, Doctor."

I was filthy, my jeans and blue work shirt wet and my hiking boots muddy. "It's 'Ben' out here on the farm."

"Please, call me Jonathan."

Frank joined us, and Domino came to the fence. We then unloaded two of the most beautiful animals I had ever seen. Compared with Domino, they were tall, their heads fine and shoulders prominent with powerful hindquarters and long legs. Domino wasn't impressed; he was agitated. He stomped and threw his head around as if he knew these mares were going to be added to his pasture. He was gelded, so they were not going to be amorous playmates—just unwanted occupants.

Jonathan explained that Mindy had visited his place, picked out these two, and worked with both briefly. "Mindy recommended the slightly taller brown mare with the blaze for Frank because she was 'a little easier to ride' and the bay for Ben because she had 'very smooth gaits but was a little difficult to handle.'"

The mares had names; Frank's was "Galla-B," and mine was "Whirley-Wee."

By now, Domino was beside himself. He scraped the ground with a front hoof, nickered, and reared up as our mares were turned loose in the pasture. What followed was the greatest show on earth: the laying back of ears, the running, rearing, kicking, and biting.

Frank asked, "Is anyone gonna get hurt?"

Jonathan shook his head. "Happens every time I bring a new horse home, and I always enjoy the show."

Finally, Domino understood he would remain king of the pasture.

My own horse! A Thoroughbred. I felt as happy as a seven-year-old with a new puppy. It was good to be a kid again.

In 1964, the term wasn't in use yet, but this was the beginning of animal-assisted therapy for one stressed-out internist.

• • •

The previous year when I took a long weekend off from Germany to visit London, I passed an equestrian shop where riding attire was on display in the window. I knew I'd be living in Maryland and had decided I would buy a Thoroughbred. I tried on a pair of full-seat breeches in tan. I was rather dashing, I thought. The shop owner, recognizing a would-be dandy, said, "Well then, sir, a hunting shirt would look very smart." He insisted I try one on. It did complement the breeches, but it was more than even my ego could stand. I could pretend to justify the breeches and future purchase of boots to prevent chafing from the stirrup straps. Being thrown was part of riding; a helmet would protect my head. Being a fop from the waist down I could handle, but not from head to toe.

• • •

Sunday morning I wore my boots, breeches, T-shirt, and hard hat. Frank and I never went to church, but even the threat of damnation could not have kept us from trying out our new mares. At first, it went well. They were easy to catch with a little feed in a bucket. Bridling was also easy enough, and the saddle did not seem to bother either mare. Frank mounted first. I hooked a lead to the bridle, and we went for an uneventful walk. We then switched to the lunge line.

All went well until Frank lightly tapped Galla-B with a crop, and he was off to the races. The same thing happened to me on Whirley-Wee. There was no concept of trot or canter; it was either walk or run.

I used the excuse of midday heat to take a nap. The riding master in Wisconsin used to say, "You ride and control a horse with your knees." I wasn't used to grabbing things with my knees, so when I woke from my nap, I was stiff but not sore enough to keep me from working Whirley-Wee until late afternoon.

• • •

My weekend had been full but so had my first full week on 2 East. Time seemed so different in my two domains.

At Kirkhill, I didn't wear a watch; that was what the sun was for, and my stomach suggested when to eat. I could enjoy the weather, be refreshed by rain, and absorb the tranquility of the setting sun. The weather outside our cabin just happened. Words could be found, put in a letter, and all this shared with Kristina.

At NIH, I parceled out time in minutes among specific tasks: history and physical exams before the dreaded bone-marrow aspiration. I also had to set priorities for things that had to be done or that I wanted to do: notes in charts, rounds; and assigned time left over to talk to my patients and their mothers, lunch with Jerry and Rick, or a trip to the library. I was aware of my own internal weather, could feel the threat of an emotional storm associated with a bone-marrow aspiration, and worried about a lightning strike of relapse or sepsis, but I didn't know how to express these emotions or share them with anyone else.

These thoughts occurred at the horses' fence, and it would be at the fence that on most nights I'd try to make sense of my day and deal with my emotions in the silence of the night.

Tired and sore, I went to bed in need of sleep to prepare for another kind of work Monday morning.

Third Week

The only name listed on the Board for me was Billy Sullivan. One-third of a triple treat: Billy, Bear, and Mrs. Sullivan.

After saying good morning to both Billy and Mrs. Sullivan, I asked, "Where's Bear?"

Billy produced Bear with a smile. I looked him over, felt his tummy, and put my stethoscope to Bear's chest, all to Billy's amusement. "Looks like Bear had a bath."

"Delicate wash in cold water, auto perm press in the dryer," Mrs. Sullivan volunteered.

I smiled. "What setting do you use for Billy?"

"It's tempting on some days," was Mrs. Sullivan's casual retort. "It's amazing how fast Billy can go from clean to dirty."

After I had obtained the interim history from Mrs. Sullivan and completed my exam, I asked, "Are you trained in one of the health-care professions? You seem to know medical terminology."

"No. My circle of 2 East friends likes to exchange information. For example, when you explained about getting the packing out of Billy's nose as soon as possible to prevent infection, I passed that on."

Then her voice dropped. "Doctor Lottsfeldt explained the toxicity of methotrexate on the oral mucosa to Linda, Jennifer's mom." She wiped a tear from one eye. "Billy and I were home, but a couple of my friends called to tell me about Jennifer."

"We all felt bad about Jennifer, Mrs. Sullivan." I sat back in my chair and swallowed hard. After a pause, I returned to the mechanics of management. "Doctor Sandler is using the treatment room. I should be able to do Billy's marrow in about thirty minutes."

I went back to the office. I'd had this problem before, when I was an intern on the pulmonary service. One of my favorite patients was an English gentleman. He had terminal emphysema and could barely walk from his bed to the sink, but he tried to accomplish this task three times a day. It was, as he said, "My Everest." On the day he died, I shared with my attending my respect and admiration for the patient and told him I was sad. He asked me to join him for a cup of coffee in his office. "You're doing a good job, and it is to your credit as a human being that you have feelings for a patient. But you're now a physician. You're going to be an internist. You need to guard against getting emotionally involved with a patient. Objectivity results in the best practice of medicine." This was a common problem for a few young doctors, he said. He was one of the professors in medicine I really liked and respected. I didn't take his comments as a reprimand; they were more a philosophical statement. I thanked him and started to leave. "Come back for another cup of coffee anytime. My door is always open."

A knock on the door. Brigid brought me back to 2 East. "Doctor Humphrey, we're ready to do Billy's marrow." As we walked down the hall, I thought, to hell with not getting emotionally involved. A little empathy for one year wouldn't ruin my academic career in internal medicine.

• • •

Tuesday afternoon, I had nothing to do until Dee told me about a new admission. "It's just for pain control and terminal care," she said. "Jimmy is a sweet, quiet boy. His mother, Mrs. Paul, is very caring, very dedicated. You know about Doctor Karon's protocol on disclosure, don't you?"

"Yes, all the patients, regardless of age, are told they have leukemia."

"The disclosure protocol started last spring. It's mandatory for all newly diagnosed patients, but when we asked mothers already under our care, most refused to allow us to tell their child the diagnosis."

"Hum. I hadn't thought about the *L* word. I was trained to always tell adults what they had."

"Mrs. Paul is opposed to Doctor Karon's program of disclosure. Very opposed. Just be prepared. He's in room six."

"Thanks, I appreciate that."

"She did want Jimmy to receive the experimental drug daunomycin," Dee said.

"Hi, Jimmy, I'm your new doctor. Doctor Billingsworth is no longer on the floor," I said. Slowly he looked up from a puzzle and gave a slight nod, no smile. A few strands of blond hair lay in disarray on a pale bald head. His blue eyes were sunken, and there was a tremor in his hand as he worked on a puzzle.

I picked up a piece. "Looks like part of a corner," I said. Again, the slow upward gaze. He took the piece, politely looked it over, laid it down, and took another.

"He's very independent, Doctor Humphrey," Mrs. Paul said.

I hadn't mentioned my name, which was bad form, but she knew it anyway. "That's obvious," I said. "Something I'll respect working with Jimmy." I liked her; she was proud of her son, respected his independence.

Mrs. Paul asked to see me for a minute out in the hall. She was dark haired, almost as tall as me, and twenty pounds heavier. She was as determined as the Berlin Wall to regulate the flow of information into Jimmy's room. "Doctor and the staff are now telling the children they have leukemia. I won't allow that; he does not know. You will not tell him."

I nodded. "I know, Mrs. Paul, and I'll be glad to honor that."

I went back to Jimmy and started to do a complete exam as was the tradition in internal medicine. Mrs. Paul held one of Jimmy's hands. I was as gentle as possible. Mrs. Paul's eyes followed my every move. Because the canal was blocked with wax, I could not see his right eardrum with the otoscope. I started to make a note to have his canal irrigated but then stopped. Who gives a rat's rump what his eardrum looks like? Irrigation hurts and could cause a bleed. If he gets a middle-ear infection, he'll tell you it hurts, and your job will be to prescribe morphine. Get with the program, dummy.

Continuing my exam, I didn't do anything that might cause pain or even discomfort, and when I was done, I helped Jimmy to a sitting position. "I won't do anything further to interrupt your work on that puzzle,"

I said and left. Later, I went back, admired his completed puzzle, and was told by his mother everything was OK.

That night at the fence, I pondered my day. My third week on 2 East, and there was going to be a third death: first Baby Boy Williams, then Jennifer Johnson, and now Jimmy Paul. I thought, it's hard to be objective under this kind of stress.

• • •

Next morning, Jimmy lay becalmed on a sea of spilled milk and cereal. Spoon at the ready, scooping up a few Cheerios with a trembling hand, he managed to get one at a time into his mouth, occasionally two. Recognizing my astonishment at his persistence, Mrs. Paul smiled. "He won't let me feed him."

I liked this duo.

After lunch, I visited Jimmy alone.

Jimmy looked around. No mom. With a direct stare, he asked, "How do kids get into heaven?"

Nothing in my training had prepared me for this question. This was not a time to discuss Huston Smith or Lao Tzu. Buying time, I walked slowly to the other side of his bed and sat in his mother's chair.

"What do you know about heaven, Jimmy?"

"That's where you go when you die." The steady stare continued.

Another ruse came to me. "Do you know anybody in heaven?"

"My grandfather."

My father sometimes answered questions by reflecting on his youth. "Well, Jimmy, when I was your age, I liked to fish with my grandfather. When he died, I knew he had gone to heaven." I paused. "I believed that when I died, I'd join him, and we'd go fishing."

The stare softened; he sank back into his pillow. I was being dismissed.

Standing in the hall, I must have been in a stupor.

"Are you all right, Doctor Humphrey?" Brigid asked.

My mind returned to 2 East. "Yes. Yes," I said, turning to recognize her question. "Everything is OK." Well, Humphrey, you kept your word. You didn't tell him he had leukemia—a stupid thought.

When Jimmy went to his heaven two days later, I reflected on his question. How sad he hadn't asked his very caring mother. She would have cried. Maybe they would have cried together.

Room 6 belonged to Jimmy. Occasionally, when I passed it, I'd think about our conversation. It didn't happen every day or every week. Just occasionally, when I was tired or my defenses were down.

• • •

A seminar on diseases, exposure to toxins, and syndromes associated with leukemia kept me in the Clinical Center until five in the evening. Nothing new. The etiology in most cases of leukemia was not known: idiopathic, as it's called in medicine. Associations included exposure to radiation therapy, immunodeficiency syndromes, and congenital anomalies such as Down syndrome. Important if a mom wants to know what causes leukemia.

After a leisurely dinner in Bethesda, I was stopping by 2 East to say hello to Billy Sullivan when I ran into Sharon, the young nurse I stressed out by asking her to check my first POMP orders. "Hi. Did you pull the evening shift this week?" I asked.

"Oh no," Sharon said with a smile. "I'm now assigned to the evening shift. It's great; I love it."

Trying to poke a little fun at myself, I quipped, "Do you mean if I want my POMP orders checked, I'll have to wait for the evening shift to start?"

Sharon laughed. "I hear you and Doctor Sandler and Doctor Lottsfeldt are doing a great job."

After Barbara told me there were no problems, I asked about Sharon.

"She readily admits she couldn't handle the screaming and crying associated with IVs and bone marrows," Barbara said. "By noon on Monday she was a nervous wreck, but she so wanted to work with our children that Dee thought it might be worth trying her here on the evening shift."

"Well, she seems to be happy," I said.

"I love having her on the floor," Barbara said. "Helping the kids at bedtime is her thing. She talks to the moms, finds out about the home bedtime routine—stories, nursery rhymes, lullabies, or prayers—and if the mom agrees, that's what she does. Now most of the toddlers don't cry themselves to sleep. I just hope it works out."

"This is a trial?"

"Doctor Humphrey, they don't *all* die during the day."

Two weeks later, Sharon took a week's leave of absence when one of Rick's patients died during the evening hours. She returned to work with children in a different unit of the Clinical Center—juvenile rheumatoid arthritis, a crippling disease. They suffer, but they too need to be sung to sleep.

● ● ●

The three of us sat down together at a quarter past two in the afternoon in the doctors' office for our Friday checkout. I was on call. Rick volunteered to take my call because of Jimmy Paul's death. I thanked him but said it wasn't necessary. Death was going to be part of some—many—most weeks, I thought. Besides, I had the horses and the fence. A place to go each evening, not to look for answers but to admit I had none.

Jerry had gone through hell with the death of a four-year-old named Wilbur Lincoln. Wilbur had died on Wednesday. Rick and I listened as Jerry described his ordeal with sepsis: the rapid onset of shock, falling blood pressure, and preterminal coma. Jerry wanted to describe in detail his attempt to console Wilbur's mom. We let Jerry take all the time he needed. Rick and I had the credentials to listen. Neither of us could think of anything of value to say, though our sympathy filled the silence of the room.

• • •

Friday night at the fence, I thought about my on-call responsibilities. Three weeks on 2 East had taught me that the nurses were a first line of defense, and Rick was a willing backup. Freireich had made it clear: "Call me anytime, day or night." Some of the mothers knew more than me, and that was OK—well, more than OK. If they could cope with leukemia full-time, I could cope with the problems of 2 East, whether they occurred during the day or when I was on call.

There was a legion of help: a good team to be part of. With that realization, I went to bed.

• • •

Up early, I let Shonto out, wolfed down a bowl of cereal, and drank a cup of coffee at the fence with the horses. I wanted to make my rounds at NIH early and be back at Kirkhill by lunchtime. Frank had asked Mindy to give us a lesson that afternoon.

Eight fifteen. Rounds were easy. First I checked in with the nurses. Barbara was in charge. She reminded me of a favorite great-aunt. I could grumble about chemotherapy to Barbara. She didn't like POMP. Barbara was a buddy but not a comrade. Bitching about Freireich was reserved for gripe sessions with Jerry and Rick.

Rick's two patients on POMP were doing well. My physical exams failed to find anything of concern. Before I wrote my note on the chart, I searched carefully for sores in the mouth.

In 1964, the Clinical Center did not have pagers. If you were on call, you signed out to a phone at home, the home of a friend, a restaurant, or wherever you'd be. If you were out shopping, you called the hospital periodically.

"Barbara, I'll be working with my horse this afternoon. I'll call in every hour."

"If you wish."

By lunchtime, I was grooming Whirly-Wee, and when Mindy arrived, I called the hospital before starting my lesson.

"Everything is fine," Barbara reported. She added, "Go sit on your horse."

Mindy wore jeans, a blue work shirt, and a baseball cap. "I can tell you've been riding tennessee walkers, Ben. Get those stirrups up where they belong."

I protested, "They're not down as if I were on a walker."

"No," said Mindy, "but they're not high enough for three-gaited." She raised each stirrup two notches.

Frank was amused. "You'll have to come back every now and then, Mindy. I enjoy seeing Ben put in his place."

Mindy and I both laughed. "You're next, Frank. Your hands are all wrong."

And so went the afternoon. We enjoyed Mindy's brisk manner and respected her knowledge. She seemed to be amused by working with two Midwestern boneheads.

After the lesson, I called 2 East. Morgan assured me everything was OK. Then Barbara got on the phone. "Doctor Humphrey, you don't have to call in so often. If anything does happen, we can take care of it for a few hours."

What a wonderful day. In the pasture at Kirkhill, I didn't know everything, and in the hospital, I just wasn't all that important.

Fourth Week

Monday mornings were now falling into a pattern. Jerry brought in a copy of the *New York Times*. The one on call gave a brief summary of the patients and new admissions. If the weekend's patient management was not complicated by problems, we talked about our private lives. When a patient had suffered significant toxicity during the weekend or a death occurred, little conversation followed.

It had been a quiet weekend, so Jerry wanted to know about my horse. I kept it simple. Jerry had never been on a horse, and Rick had only taken a few pony rides. I tried to regale them with the joy of working a green horse. On this Monday morning, I was sore and stiff from too much riding. I told them, "Today will be a sitting-down-slowly day."

Jerry shook his head. "How could any normal male want to get dirty, shovel manure, risk life and limb, and get a sore *tuchis* when the bars of Georgetown are full of eager women? One of these days, I'm gonna fix you up with someone."

"I assume that *tuchis* means butt," Rick said.

Jerry and I applauded.

Morgan came in with the list of new patients. I forgot what she told the other two. "I have bad news for you, Doctor H. You have three admissions—all nice kids and very good mothers," she said.

"Hey, I'll take one of the three off your hands, Ben," Jerry said.

Rick shrugged. "I can do it, Jerry, if you've got something planned for this evening,"

"Hey, guys. Thanks, three admissions might keep me on 2 East for an extra two hours, but I don't need to be home early enough to ride." I reminded them, "I have a *tuchis* problem."

• • •

Three admissions! It was going to be a long day. I didn't care about the hours. I had now been on 2 East for three weeks, so I no longer minded writing chemotherapy orders using the body surface area. I knew from experience that it was the three bone-marrow aspirations and three venipunctures that were going to wipe me out.

Rick and Jerry suggested I do my marrows first. They'd write their admission notes while I used the treatment room. They pointed out that I'd need both Morgan and Brigid.

Both nurses were way ahead of me.

"Doctor H., I'll introduce you to each mother and explain the need for a brief history and a limited physical exam," Morgan said.

"I'll go to the treatment room and get three marrow trays ready," Brigid said. "Morgan, you and I can take turns bringing the child to the treatment room and doing the holding during the marrow."

"Thanks. I don't know which is worse: bringing a crying child to the treatment room or listening to their screams while holding them down," Morgan said.

"Monday morning is pure hell until I look at the marrow up in the path lab. I like telling a mom there are no leukemia cells."

An hour later the crying, screaming, and breaking of little bones was all over. All three aspirates failed to reveal any leukemia cells; all three patients were in remission. I wrote three sets of orders for POMP. Wearing my best professional facade, I refused to let the emotional turmoil of the morning rise to the surface.

After that, I could slow down, relax, and spend time with my patients and their mothers. The best part of Monday morning.

• • •

Brigid had suggested I start with Tammy Long, a ten-year-old. Mrs. Long and Tammy were quiet. They were from a rural area of West Virginia, and Brigid was of the opinion that this large health-care facility frightened the mother. "Mrs. Long gets most of her information from other mothers and the nurses and seldom asks questions of the doctor. I like her; you'll like Tammy."

OK, I thought. Mrs. Long and I are both intimidated by the Clinical Center. And why not? It had taken me two weeks to find the library from

2 East without getting lost. The building was a block long, and there were two parallel halls in the long axis as well as two wings. If it hadn't been for the "You Are Here" signs at each elevator, each set of stairs, and most corners, I might have starved to death somewhere in this labyrinth.

A rather large child, Tammy sat next to her mother. She wore an auburn wig. On her bed were several fashion magazines and an older-looking stuffed doll that had apparently survived six or seven years of loving. She had been in remission for several months, and the vincristine part of POMP had resulted in complete hair loss.

After two or three courses of POMP, every patient was bald. The volunteers had a supply of free wigs. All the patients I had encountered during the first three weeks on 2 East couldn't be bothered because wigs were hot. Baseball caps for the boys and colored scarves for the girls were cooler.

Mrs. Long was of average height. The skin of her face and hands had a weathered look. Her hair was light brown with a few strands of premature gray. Her makeup was simple: only lipstick. She wore a light-yellow dress and no jewelry except a thin gold wedding band.

My first few noninvasive questions were answered with a nod or a shake of the head. I got a chair and sat down. I thought my standing over Mrs. Long and Tammy might account for the short answers. Sitting would suggest I wasn't in a hurry, but Mrs. Long continued to either nod or use monosyllabic responses.

When I tried to engage Tammy in conversation, she would turn and look at her mother. She took off her wig.

"Tammy wanted to make a good impression on her new doctor," Mrs. Long said.

"Tammy, you're a pretty girl with or without the wig!" For a young girl, fashion and looking pretty was important. Tammy had accomplished her mission.

Outside in the hall, I organized my notes and then thought, if you live in or near a very small town where there's no hospital and your only health-care experience is at a doctor's office, what's it like to come to this campus and its Clinical Center?

• • •

Brigid suggested I see Michelle Karr next. "She's a real treat. One of the sweetest babies we have on the floor."

Interesting, I thought. I liked every little patient I had come in contact with, even Sarah Thompkins, who didn't like me.

Sitting on Mrs. Karr's ample lap was a chubby bald one-year-old. Mrs. Karr wasn't overweight; she was obese. She had a round face and short curly hair and wore a loose-fitting smock. Mrs. Karr was easy to interview but very soft-spoken.

Michelle looked like a model for Gerber baby foods. She kept me under a steady wide-eyed gaze. Her crib side rails were down. The bed was cluttered with a pink blanket, a blue teddy bear, a rattle, a miniature rocking horse with a rooster on each end, and a circular teething ring.

When I pulled my chair forward to listen to Mrs. Karr, Michelle extended her arms.

"May I pick her up?"

"Of course," Mrs. Karr smiled. "Two of the nurses have already been in and had Michelle on their laps. This is our third admission. I guess Michelle is sort of a mascot."

I had to swallow hard. Internal medicine is a lapless specialty.

Mrs. Karr said Michelle had never sat on Doctor Billingsworth's lap. She quickly added, "But Doctor B never sat down."

I did the first part of my exam with Michelle in my lap; I finished the rest of her exam on her mother's lap. Michelle never cried.

As an internist now three weeks on this pediatric unit, I was beginning to learn a few things. Whenever possible, sit down. If the baby wants to be picked up, pick up the baby and put the baby on your lap. That's what babies are for; that's what laps are for. I dubbed Michelle my "snuggle bunny."

• • •

Finally, there was Todd Yardley, a six-year-old. "Nice kid. All you have to do is break the ice," Brigid said.

Todd was sitting in bed in the lotus position. He was also bald from chemotherapy. He looked me over, neither smiling nor frowning. His bed was a jumble of plastic models of various breeds of dogs and several books about dogs.

"Give me five," I said, extending my open hand. He gave me a moderate slap, but the ice was not broken.

"This is your new doctor, Todd," Mrs. Yardley said in a reassuring tone. Todd nodded; that was all.

I could get to this six-year-old but would have to figure out how.

Mrs. Yardley was articulate. It went with her modern-librarian look. Her hair was pulled back; she wore horn-rimmed glasses and had a book in hand.

Todd was polite and cooperative but also cautious. After all, I had just done a marrow aspirate on him this morning. Finally, I said, "I just got a horse. Do you have a pet?"

"Yes!" He sat up. "My dog, Ralph."

"Ralph?"

Mrs. Yardley explained, "Todd had had an imaginary friend named Ralph, and when the dog came into our home as a puppy, there was a transmigration of a soul."

"Ralph can sit, shake hands, and sort of roll over. I teached him that," Todd said, interrupting his mother.

After his mother gently corrected Todd's grammar, I asked, "Do you have any pictures of Ralph?"

Todd pulled an envelope from under the covers. I sat on Todd's bed as we shared a photographic history of friendship. There were pictures of Ralph as a puppy with Todd when he had a full head of hair and others taken later when Ralph looked full-grown and Todd was bald. I was given a full description of each photo, and Mrs. Yardley didn't interrupt at Todd's occasional grammatical errors.

• • •

I went to the coffee shop and grabbed a sandwich and a cup of coffee. I walked outside to my bench in the shade. After the trauma of Monday's bone-marrow aspirations, I needed to rest and relax. This was the same bench I went to after the death of Baby Boy Williams.

I loosened my tie, unbuttoned my shirt at the neck, looked at the sky, noticed a few white clouds, and felt a warm breeze. If POMP didn't kill anyone or cause life-threatening toxicity, it should be a great week. There would be vomiting, of course. I fantasized about hanging up a new sign at the entrance of 2 East: "Vomiting Center."

A squirrel scampered down from the tree and begged for a bit of my lunch. On such a good day, he got a corner of my sandwich. He downed it quickly; I didn't know squirrels liked tuna.

"Well, little buddy, I guess I'd better start bringing a bag of nuts with me when I come to this bench. I'm going to name you Squirrel. Let me tell you about a dog named Ralph."

• • •

The IVs were all started by half past two. I returned to each room for a nontraumatic visit before chemotherapy began. Bad enough for them to remember me as the guy who stuck them with needles. I didn't want to reinforce that I was also the guy making them vomit.

Tammy and her mother were looking at a magazine together. Mrs. Long frowned.

"This is just a social call. Do you have any questions?"

She smiled. "You stop by anytime you wish, Doctor."

When I entered Todd's room, his mother closed the book she was reading and asked, "What's wrong, Doctor Humphrey?"

"Nothing's wrong, Mrs. Yardley. I just stopped by to ask if you had any questions, and it's also my chance to hear another story about Ralph."

"You startled me. Doctor Billingsworth only came in during the afternoon if there was a problem. Todd will never run out of stories about Ralph. You two go ahead and talk about dogs. I'm also a dog lover, especially when it comes to Ralph."

So that was why Mrs. Long frowned at my appearance. I'd have to demonstrate to these moms that I wasn't Doctor Billingsworth.

Michelle was not in her room. I went to the nurses' station to write on the three charts. There, sitting on Morgan's lap, was Michelle.

• • •

After dinner in the cafeteria, I drove to Kirkhill at dusk. The day was over. A one-year-old named Michelle had reached out to me, a seven-year-old named Tammy had worn a hot wig so she would look good when we met, and a six-year-old named Todd had a special friend named Ralph. It had been a day of trauma, but I had met three nice little people. Images of these three flashed before me. I was bonding with three more patients again.

I was tired and exhausted but happy. Keep on asking, I thought, what do I need to know to take good care of these little patients?

• • •

Breaking Little Bones

The drive in to NIH was refreshing top-down weather. When I walked onto 2 East, I imagined all was well. I checked in with the nurses; all three IVs I had started yesterday were running. All three patients' names were on the Board without red ink. Morgan handed me my charts. There was something in her smile that suggested the vital signs and laboratory data were all OK. None of my patients had a fever, and none complained about a sore mouth.

Freireich showed up at exactly 10:00 a.m. The three of us were ready. With a keen eye, he prowled through charts and laboratory data. He was satisfied; all the patients were on schedule. Jay said he didn't have any questions. He was off the floor in twenty minutes, and we were glad to be rid of him.

At a quarter past eleven, I went to the library's large table where the newest issues of various journals were displayed and picked up copies of the *Journal of Biochemistry, Journal of the American Medical Association,* and the *Annals of Internal Medicine.* I sat down and sighed.

There would be other mornings, afternoons, evenings, and weekends like this throughout the year. It wouldn't always be screams, tears, and the Board full of red ink.

• • •

POMP-associated toxicity was either happening or we were waiting for it to happen. In the library, I was acquiring a grim idea of the influence of each of the four drugs on bone-marrow function.

Billy Sullivan had taught me about the platelets. They were the smallest particles that could be seen with a light microscope, and the normal number per cubic millimeter of blood was two hundred thousand. A moderate suppression of their number—say one hundred thousand—was not associated with bleeding, but below twenty thousand, bleeding did occur. POMP therapy turned off platelet production, and the lowest platelet count tended to occur halfway between courses of therapy. Platelet recovery occurred during the second half of the time off therapy.

Jerry's case of fatal sepsis from the previous week was an example of one of the most feared toxicities. Very low numbers of white blood cells were associated with fever—either a viral infection or bacteria growing rapidly in the bloodstream. One couldn't tell one cause of fever from the other, so all patients with a low white-blood-cell count and fever had blood drawn for cultures, and IV antibiotics were given. If the blood cultures remained sterile, with no growth, and the patient remained without fever for a day or two, we assumed it was a virus; IV antibiotics were stopped and the patient sent home. If a bacterium did grow in the blood cultures, it was characterized, its sensitivity to various antibiotics was determined, and optimal therapy continued for ten days. In many cases, ten days of antibiotic therapy prevented fatal sepsis.

On Wednesday afternoon, Todd spiked a fever. I explained all this to Mrs. Yardley. She already knew about the uncertainty of a fever in a child receiving chemotherapy.

"It's a different kind of limbo," she said.

This was a short-term threat to her son's life that Todd would overcome.

• • •

Friday morning at a quarter past eleven, we sat together to discuss any patients who were not going home. Rick was on call. Jerry for once didn't have any patients with clinically significant toxicity. I discussed Todd. He had spiked only the one fever on Wednesday. Todd's blood cultures were still sterile, so I hoped for the best. Rick had one patient receiving chemotherapy.

As I came back from lunch at half past one, I met Mrs. Long and Tammy leaving 2 East. Mrs. Long nudged Tammy, who came forward and said, "Thank you, Doctor Humphrey." Mrs. Long added, "I hope you have a pleasant weekend riding your horse." I hadn't mentioned Whirley-Wee, but Mrs. Yardley must have told them.

Mrs. Karr told me she had learned from Kathryn Sullivan, Billy's mom, about the advice I'd given to her about nose care to reduce bleeding. "Good ideas," she said and then added that she talked to Kathryn "all the time."

For scientists, the exchange is called the literature; for clinical associates, a bull session; and for mothers, a network. When talking to a mom, there is only one way to explain something. Don't try to protect one mom with a little lie and then tell another the truth because you think she can take it.

On 2 East, we had a rule. No matter how bad the answer, there was only one: the truth.

• • •

Saturday morning called for blue jeans. I saddle soaped my tack. Frank was mowing the lawn, so I cleaned his tack too. A fair exchange, I thought. My work was done in shade: quiet, clean work. Then grooming. I liked the smell of a horse far better than grass clippings.

Afternoon was for riding britches, the lunge line, the saddle, and the bridle. It was walk, walk, and walk. Under a July sun, I thought, walking was cool, while running was work. At present, Whirley-Wee didn't have "the brains God gave a goose," as one of my great aunts was wont to say. Five, ten, maybe fifteen minutes of walking, and then there was head shaking, a nicker or two, and a little prance, as if she were trying to say, "Let's get at it. I was bred to run."

I would stop her in her tracks and say, "I'm a control freak. We're going to walk some more. We'll run another day." Whirley-Wee was a beautiful animal. I wanted a well-trained, responsive horse. So we would work on walking. "This is not a waste of time. We'll do some walking on rides, and we'll walk when you need to cool down."

Morning chores, midday focus on the horse, and a refreshing late-afternoon shower. Before my evening meal, I couldn't keep away from the phone any longer. "Barbara, this is Doctor Humphrey. How is Todd?"

"He's fine, Doctor Humphrey. No growth on the blood cultures. Doctor Lottsfeldt plans to stop the antibiotics tomorrow. Now you relax; everything's OK!"

"I'm sorry to have bothered you, Barbara. I just wanted to know."

"That's all right. I'm getting used to you. And Doctor Sandler. And Doctor Lottsfeldt."

I hung up and thought, what the hell? That was what phones were for, and it only took a couple of minutes. Besides, Barbara liked to grumble.

The first month was over. To the best of my knowledge, I hadn't killed anyone. I'd been short-tempered and wasn't going to let that happen again. I had survived thanks to the camaraderie of Rick and Jerry, a bevy of nurses, and a host of mothers.

AUGUST

First Week

The second cycle of my patients was about to begin, and I was pleased to renew my acquaintance with the first week's pair from July. Both names were on the Board.

Sarah Thompkins, my six-year-old with her Barbie dolls, didn't like me, but I liked her honesty. John Graham, eleven years old, with abdominal obstruction from a lymphoma, was another matter. Because he had suffered through the nausea and vomiting of POMP, he had withdrawn.

Seeing me in the hall, Dee approached. "Doctor Humphrey, Mrs. Graham wants to see you before you examine John. I'll tell her you're here."

"Good morning, Doctor Humphrey," Mrs. Graham said in her usual cordial manner. We walked down to the doctors' office. After closing the door and suggesting that she sit down, I had to ask.

"Is John vomiting again? Is he complaining of abdominal pain?"

"Oh no. I just wanted to explain about the drawing of the tumor in the belly. That approach didn't work. I didn't want to tell you in front of John. I don't want him to feel I'm disappointed in his behavior."

My shoulder relaxed.

"When we got home, I explained the use of the drawings to my husband. He suggested that we give John a few days to adjust to being home before doing the drawing. My husband must've sensed something was wrong."

"Was John happy to be home?"

"Not really. And two days later, when I got out the drawing paper, John wouldn't participate. His dad said, 'We don't have to do this today.'"

"Did you try again?"

"Yes. A week later. This time with my younger sister, John's favorite aunt. As soon as she got the drawing pad out, he yelled no and ran out of the room. John doesn't want to talk or do anything with anyone."

I shook my head and tried to sort out my feelings: sadness, disappointment, and sorrow. After a minute, I said, "I'm sorry the drawing caused so much stress."

"We have a senior pediatric oncologist, Doctor Karon, on the staff," I said. "I'll go ask if he can help with this problem."

• • •

Down the hall, when I asked Sarah how she was doing, Mrs. Thompkins answered for her daughter, "We're gettin' on." Mrs. Thompkins seemed more at ease with me this time, speaking more spontaneously. The interim history that she gave was unremarkable. When I finished, Mrs. Thompkins asked, "Is John Graham already here?"

"Yes."

"Julia Graham and me got real close last month. It was a bad time for her after John went home. That drawing about puking."

I opened the door for Mrs. Thompkins. She walked out into the hall and found Mrs. Graham waiting. They embraced and spoke softly, as two sisters might. Most of the conversation flowed from Mrs. Thompkins to Mrs. Graham.

That's an odd friendship, I thought. Mary Sue Thompkins probably played bingo at church once a week, while Julia Graham was more likely to play bridge at a country club.

• • •

Our weekly morning rounds with Freireich should have been simple. I presented John Graham to Freireich. After reminding him of the tumor obstruction, the radiotherapy, and the first course of POMP, I commented that on physical exam I couldn't feel anything in his abdomen and asked if he wanted an upper-GI barium study to determine the size of any residual tumor.

"No," said Freireich. "As long as he's clinically responding, just give him monthly courses of chemotherapy. He's not an evaluable patient for the POMP protocol, so there's no reason to put him through an unnecessary procedure."

Freireich must have seen the astonishment on my face. "Look, Ben, POMP is limited to patients with acute lymphocytic leukemia or ALL, not patients with lymphomas. Lymphomas need something different: radiation, plus some kind of chemotherapy. I have a feeling from the literature that an alkylating agent like cyclophosphamide should be added to any lymphoma regimen."

"Sir," I said, "why was he admitted to 2 East? John's going through hell with the bone marrows, IV therapy, and vomiting."

Jerry sat up straight, and Rick went so far as to say, "I don't understand."

"Lymphomas, also called lymphosarcomas, occur in the GI tract or abdomen, the mediastinum or neck, and in lymph nodes," Freireich said. "Some of these cases can have circulating malignant cells in the blood at diagnosis."

"Is that what's meant by a leukemic conversion in a patient who presents with a lymphoma?" Jerry asked.

"Yes. But sometimes you can get tricked into thinking a case is leukemia when it's a lymphoma. Herbert Wollner runs an office that screens patient referrals. He took the call on Graham, a patient who was thought to have leukemia cells in his blood. By the time Graham got here, he was almost completely obstructed. I could feel a mass in his abdomen. Graham's peripheral blood did contain immature lymphocytes like you can see in a viral infection, but there were no leukemia cells. Graham needed to be treated. He was sick, and it's our policy not to send patients back home if they have cancer."

• • •

When I called Myron about John Graham, he told me, "Stop by anytime today." Myron had a philosophical way of looking at some things that was refreshing. He listened to the course of John Graham's treatment and his current state of withdrawal.

"That's a bit unusual, Ben. To not relate to you as a physician—that's common. But to withdraw from family support—that's uncommon. You know about our disclosure protocol, telling all patients the name of their disease. You've already told John that he has a lymphoma, so I'll ask our social worker to spend some time with John. Joel's very good; he may learn something."

"Good idea! I'm sure Mrs. Graham will appreciate that her concern is being taken seriously."

"I'm glad you think it's important. You know that's not bad for an egghead like you. There may be hope for you yet," Myron said with a smile.

I enjoyed his gibe. "You're a son of a bitch."

"I'm called a 'dumb son of a bitch' by laboratory-oriented staff."

"Oh?"

"We're just beginning to look into these types of problems. This type of inquiry is called psychosocial bullshit. I take a lot of crap about the disclosure protocol. It's not science, they say. Thank God I've got Jay's support."

Myron was way ahead of his time.

• • •

Wednesday, 9:00 a.m. Time for the scheduled monthly lecture. In July, Jay Freireich had reviewed the development of drug trials in leukemia. While these were empirical trials, I had to admit there had been progress in prolonging remissions despite the lack of any theoretical considerations.

In the medical literature, the lecturer was known as Emil Frei III; we called him Tom. Tall, thin, and handsome, he wore metal-rimmed glasses. Tom was articulate and erudite. He showed slides depicting intermediate metabolism, drawings of the structure of molecules, graphs, tables of data, and some statistics. I was enthralled, but I heard a low groan from Jerry.

Possible chemotherapy in ALL began with research on folic acid, a member of the vitamin B complex. When given to patients with leukemia, it stimulates leukemia-cell growth. Doctor Sidney Farber, working with children with leukemia at Harvard, had asked Doctor Y. SubbaRow from Lederle Laboratories to synthesize the first antagonist of folic acid, aminopterin. When this agent was given to sixteen terminally ill patients, ten went into a temporary complete remission. "In 1948, these results were published in the *New England Journal of Medicine*," Tom said. As an aside he added, "This major advance was ridiculed by some physicians. Some of us now consider Farber to be the father of cancer chemotherapy."

The next advance in rational drug design began in 1945 with two chemists, George Hitchings and Gertrude Elion, who were working at the Burroughs Wellcome Company. Adenine is a building block of DNA. Tom explained, "The adenine molecule is contains an amino group, $-H_2N$, and when that is replaced a thio group, $=S$, the resulting molecule is 6-mercaptopurine, or 6-MP, which blocks DNA synthesis."

Tom went on. "Doctor Joseph Burchenal, at Memorial Sloan-Kettering Cancer Center in New York, decided to try the same antimetabolite approach to treating leukemia as Farber had pioneered with folic-acid antagonists. In 1953, a clinical trial of 6-MP in patients resistant to methotrexate resulted in one-third of those individuals going into remission."

G. Bennett Humphrey

I had studied the structure of biological molecules as a graduate student in biochemistry and was fascinated with this chemistry of rational drug research. What interested me was that 6-mercaptopurine and aminopterin do not occur in nature; these molecules were made in the lab. By chemically altering one small area of a larger normal biological molecule, chemists created man-made drugs that killed cancer cells.

Doctor Frei's historical review of vincristine was short. The anticancer activity of this drug was an accidental finding. Pharmacologists at Eli Lilly were screening plant alkaloids for antidiabetic activity. Vincristine isolated from the madagascar-periwinkle plant was observed to block the proliferation of tumor cells. Given to patients with ALL as a single agent, vincristine will induce a remission 50 percent of the time. These studies were reported in the early 1960s.

The last class of drugs presented by Tom was the corticosteroids. Prednisone and related drugs were known to influence lymphocytes. The use of this group of drugs in the treatment of leukemia reported a 50 percent remission induction in 1949.

The three of us rode the elevator down to 2 East. Rick knew a bit of the recent history of drug development in leukemia. "You know, when Jay and Tom first started to combine all four drugs in 1962, we were severely criticized, even accused of torturing children."

• • •

Not all of my patients were hospitalized. As clinical associates of the National Cancer Institute, we spent most of our time on 2 East, also known as the inpatient service. Occasionally patients were scheduled to be seen in the outpatient department (OPD). Long-term follow-up was an oxymoron in the 1960s—except for Carl Shively.

An OPD nurse called to tell me of my appointment with Carl and suggested that I come early to review his chart. "He's a very unusual case," she said.

The appointment was for 2:00 p.m. I arrived at 1:15 p.m. to read Billingsworth's last note on Carl.

June 24, 1964.

> *Carl Shively has never relapsed. He has been in remission since February 1961. His remission was induced with prednisone, and his maintenance therapy has been daily oral 6-MP. Of the twenty-eight patients entered into this treatment schedule, all have died except Carl. Doctor Freireich and I reviewed Carl's response to therapy in March of this year with Mrs. Shively. The following was stressed: no one knew if the 6-MP was necessary to keep Carl in remission, and no one knew if the 6-MP could be stopped. Mrs. Shively agreed to the following plan: Carl would continue on 6-MP, but instead of monthly follow-up visits, we would see him for evaluation every other month.*
>
> > *Plan for the next year: if Carl continues in remission, review his chart with Doctor Freireich in March 1965 and again decide whether to continue maintenance 6-MP therapy.*
>
> *Dx: ALL in remission*
> *Rx: OPD follow-up every other month. Daily oral 6-MP*
>
> *John Billingsworth, MD*

The correspondence section was very interesting. Several pathologists at other institutions had reviewed the original bone marrow. All consultants diagnosed ALL. Several research oncologists at major centers were asked their opinion on continuing therapy. There was no uniform opinion, but all consultants agreed there was no definitive clinical data to justify stopping or discontinuing therapy. Good old Freireich, I thought. Internationally known for his research in leukemia, and yet, he wasn't afraid to ask for help.

Carl and his mother were on time for their appointment. "Glad to meet you, Doc. Carl, go shake hands with your new doctor," Mrs. Shively said. She was plump; a full round face sat directly on her shoulders. She had no neck, or waistline, or any break in the outline of her spheroidal torso. Mrs. Shively lacked inhibitions; what occurred to her came out unedited. There was no need for any medical persona for this pair; just be yourself, I thought.

Mrs. Shively provided an interim history of the last two months. Carl's physical exam was normal; without any instruction, he rolled over and grasped the edge of the table in preparation for the marrow aspiration. He didn't say a word until I sucked out the marrow, and then he yelled.

"I've told Carl he's got the right to scream," his mother said as she went to him and rubbed his shoulders. "It's all over, Son. You're a tough little boy, and I'm proud of you."

I returned from the path lab with the good news that the marrow was normal. I found Carl reading a comic book and his mother ready with an unrestrained observation.

"You're the fourth clinical associate that we have had, and God willing, we'll have a fifth next year." Then her voice dropped. "The others in Carl's group are all gone. He's the only one left. After each trip to this clinic, I talk to five other mothers whose kids are gone. They want to know if Carl's OK. And you know something, Doctor Humphrey? They may cry over their own loss, but they rejoice in Carl's good fortune. They're not jealous. No, sir." She wiped her eyes with the back of her hand. "I love every one of 'em. They're strong, good women, Doctor." Now tears were streaming down her cheeks. She looked up at me and smiled.

That evening I pondered this remarkable mother. All of my role models in medicine when I was a student and resident were reserved. Here was Mrs. Shively, open and in contact with her emotions.

• • •

On Friday afternoon, I was able to leave NIH by a quarter past four. Frank was having a few guests out to Kirkhill. He wanted to show off his Thoroughbred. A social gathering might do me some good, I thought.

When I arrived home, Frank was frantically preparing Italian delicacies for the evening. He had spent several evenings reading Italian cookbooks and the better part of two days cruising through food stores. I would have gladly helped but knew from experience cooking was Frank's thing, so I volunteered to groom Galla-B and get Domino ready in case any guest wanted to ride.

With the currycomb, I brought a shine to Galla-B's coat, using water and then wiping her hooves with neat's-foot oil. God, she was beautiful.

From the beauty to the clown: one did not groom Domino but just dusted him off. He was an easy pony to be around, although he would move this way or that just to be ornery. I enjoyed his capers. Besides, a well-groomed Domino would be out of character, a Huckleberry Finn in an altar boy's robe. Domino was perfect au naturel.

As the guests arrived, I met them outside, introduced myself, and suggested they admire Frank's Thoroughbred before going into the cabin. Among the guests was a single blonde named Joan. She was tastefully dressed in slacks and a short-sleeved sweater that revealed a smashing figure. She moved easily among the guests, chatting, shaking hands with some, and giving social hugs to others. She introduced herself to me and said she'd like to ride Domino after the younger guests had had their turn.

A few guests rode Domino. Joan was the last to ride and complained that the pony didn't want to trot. I suggested he might be tired and should be put back in the pasture.

Joan made herself useful by holding Domino while I put his tack away. We spent the next part of the evening talking of this and that. She was recently divorced, lived in Bethesda, and had a four-year-old son. This was her free weekend as her ex-husband was caring for their child. We arranged to have dinner Sunday night.

The next evening, we went to the Crab House on Bethesda Avenue. The atmosphere was casual, with paper on the table, and the red crabs were served with a wooden mallet, a small knife, and a lot of napkins. I liked the place, and if the conversation failed, one could spend the evening whacking open crabs.

We exchanged the information typical of a couple just beginning to date. She wanted to know all about living in Europe. After dinner, we walked. She took my arm. "I'm told European women like to walk arm in arm."

Joan was affectionate and pleasant company, but we only had a few dates.

What terminated this affair, I couldn't say. I was beginning to be aware that 2 East was consuming most of my emotional energy.

Second Week

During the previous month, I dreaded Monday mornings, but today I would get to listen to Sally Carter, my charming chatterbox. In July, I had gone to a children's bookstore and read through a book on *The Flintstones*, so I now knew most of these cartoon characters, especially Pebbles.

"I had a quiet weekend call," Jerry said. "Rick, your patient finished POMP on Sunday. Another patient of mine is on IV antibiotics, and the blood cultures remained no growth. And this week, Betty Miller will be admitted."

"The little girl who likes to sit in the hall and smiles and waves at everybody?" Rick asked.

"That's the one."

"I've got the great news," Rick said, grinning. "It is now official: my wife, Jody, is pregnant. The due date is the middle of March."

"Hey, tomorrow, you and Jody will be our guests for dinner at the officers' club across the street in the Bethesda Naval Hospital," Jerry exclaimed.

"Great idea. I'll phone her."

Jerry talked briefly of his exploits in the bars of Georgetown.

Not mentioning my date with Joan, I commented on Whirley-Wee's learning to trot.

Our friendship now included friendly personality profiles. Jerry liked to be the man about town. I was into horses, and Rick was the father-to-be. These ideas about ourselves would be used for jokes, sarcastic remarks, or dismissive statements like "What'd you expect from Ben? He prefers horses to women," "Jerry, you look spent, like you need some vitamin E," and "Well, Rick's an expectant father; they act like that."

• • •

Rick and I were outside the nurses' station looking at the Board when a little voice cried, "Doctor Humpfee." Sally, carrying Pebbles, ran down the hall ahead of her mother. She came up and gave me a hug. A great hug. Getting down on one knee, I could be eye to eye, smiling.

"Good mornin', Doctor Humphrey," Mrs. Carter said when she caught up with her daughter. She took Sally by the hand and calmly told her it was Monday. She looked at the Board and said, "Doctor Humphrey will be busy today. Tomorrow there'll be time to talk." They walked down the hall with Morgan to Sally's room.

Still kneeling, I looked up at Rick and said, "Within an hour I'm going to stick a needle into her marrow. Before lunch, I'll stick a needle into a vein. Then POMP's gonna make her vomit."

Now Rick's smile broadened. It wasn't his "I'm going to have to work with this clown for a year?" smile. It was different. More like a "maybe someday you'll understand" smile.

Tears almost came to my eyes. A three-year-old had breached the internist's palisade.

• • •

R ick came into the office. "Ben, would you do me a favor?"
"Of course."

"Will you start an IV on Vicki, a three-year-old?" Rick asked.

"Yes, of course." I frowned.

"Thanks. It's a sort of rule we used in Minnesota," Rick explained when seeing my wrinkled brow. "If you can't get an IV started in three sticks, stop and ask someone else to try. After three sticks you lose it; you lose something. You might try a foot first. I struck out on her arms."

The veins of the foot, I thought. An image from *Grey's Anatomy* came back to me: parallel veins on the top of the foot that joined an arching vein. As a freshman medical student, I probably knew the Latin names, but now only the image remained—obviously far more important.

"We're all set. Come on, Ben," Rick said. "I'll introduce you to Vicki's mom."

In the treatment room, I removed the plastic sheet and warm towel from one of Vicki's feet. After applying the tourniquet, I could feel a pulse in Vicki's foot. A thin blue line appeared. The brown color of iodine was removed with alcohol. Brigid restrained Vicki's trunk. Morgan knew exactly how to hold and immobilize a wiggling foot. She rested both of her forearms on the table, wrapping one hand around the ankle and holding both the heel and toes with the other, giving me free access to the vein. Then a phenomenon occurred that's hard to explain. The screaming continued, but I could not hear it. The wiggling of Vicki's torso went on, but I did not see it. Morgan's hands disappeared. Vicki disappeared. The whole world was a small patch of skin with a thin blue line. Blood with the first stick, and the screaming, the two nurses, and Vicki returned.

I explained the rule of three to Vicki's mom. "Everybody hates this IV therapy: the patients, the moms, the nurses, and the doctors. Doctor Lottsfeldt recommended that I try the foot, which was a good choice, and I was lucky in finding a vein."

At lunch, we discussed the rule of three. We all agreed it made walking onto the ward a little easier in the morning. All three of us exchanged stories of how we learned to start IVs on patients; some of these memories were not pleasant.

It was time for some black humor. I aped a psychiatrist starting an IV. "Now, Mr. Smith, you're withholding your veins from me. That's very juvenile behavior for a man your age."

"Maybe you had trouble with toilet training, Mr. Smith," Jerry added.

I asked, "As a young boy, did you want to sleep with your mother, Mr. Smith?"

"We're gonna have to give you electric shock treatment," Rick added.

We enjoyed a couple more exchanges, on a roll again.

• • •

Sally Carter told me of her adventures with her friend Betsy. A stream of words, phrases, and sentences flowed. Sometimes, she'd ask a question like, "Do you know what we did?"

And before I could say no, Sally would answer the question.

When I asked if Sally carried on like this at home, Mrs. Carter said, "Most of the day."

"I brought a puzzle, Doctor Humpfee," Sally told me as she pulled out a small board from her toy bag.

"We understand when you have the time, you put puzzles together here on the ward," Mrs. Carter said in her easygoing manner. "I told Sally you might help, but only if there was time."

Looking first at the puzzle, then Sally, and finally Mrs. Carter, I said, "Six pieces—that's going to be difficult. It's a good thing I took Advanced Puzzles 401. OK, let's get the plastic wrapper off."

"Are you sure you're not too busy, Doctor Humphrey?" Mrs. Carter asked.

"Time with your daughter is time well spent. She brightens my day, Mrs. Carter."

• • •

Rick and I were writing admitting notes when Jerry walked in the office and sat down with a resounding thump.

I put my pen down. "What's the matter, Jerry?"

"What makes you think there's something wrong?"

"That's the way you sat down on the day Wilbur died," I said.

"I'm sorry, Ben. You're right. I'm concerned about Betty Miller. I need to talk to you two."

Rick's chair squeaked as he turned to face Jerry.

"I'm supposed to start POMP on her today, and she's hypoplastic," Jerry said. "There are virtually no white blood cells in her blood. In her marrow—no leukemic cells—no granulocyte precursors."

Rick put out his hand, and Jerry gave him the lab slip. "We would have never given chemotherapy to a patient with counts like these in Minnesota," Rick said as he shook his head.

"Remember what Freireich said about Minnesota," I said.

"Yeah—but I don't ever want to see another Jennifer Johnson," Rick said.

• • •

On this floor of ever-present malignancy, rounds with Freireich this second week in August weren't benign.

"How's Sally Carter, Ben?" Jay asked.

"Sally's bone marrow was good, and POMP started yesterday."

"Jerry. Betty Miller?" Jay asked.

"Her blood counts were very low, especially her white count. Betty's marrow's hypoplastic—very hypoplastic—but there were no leukemic blasts present. I started her on POMP yesterday. I'm concerned about giving POMP in the presence of a marrow that hasn't recovered."

"Doctor Sandler, I look at the clinical data on all admissions. Then I compare that data to the clinical course: no fever, fever but no sepsis, fever with sepsis, death due to sepsis, and so on. So far there's no correlation with the admitting white count and sepsis."

"I'm still worried," Jerry said.

"No one is going to relapse because you're worried." Then Jay looked at Rick. "Where's Georgia Simpson's chart, Rick?"

"Everything's OK, but I thought I heard rales in her lungs. So she's in radiology getting a chest x-ray. I'll let you know if she has pneumonia," Rick said.

Rounds were over in fifteen minutes. Jay returned to his office to mull over clinical data: Jerry played a waving game with Betty, I enjoyed a story from Sally, and Rick went to radiology to look at Georgia's normal chest x-ray.

• • •

Wednesday morning, Betty was on duty at her post in the hall. Wednesday afternoon at 2:20 p.m., Betty stopped waving, and at 3:00 p.m. she spiked a fever. By 3:15 p.m. Jerry had cultured her blood and urine and written antibiotic orders.

"I know you're on call, Ben, but I asked the nurses to call me tonight if anything changes in Betty's condition," Jerry said. "I hope you don't mind."

"Of course not."

We were standing outside the nurses' station.

The hall down by Betty's room was empty.

• • •

Thursday morning, seven thirty. "How's Betty?" I entered the nurses' station and stopped myself. "I'm sorry. Let's start all over. Good morning, Brigid, I hope you're fine. How's Betty this morning?"

"Good morning, Doctor Humphrey. You don't have to apologize for worrying about Betty. She still has a fever. Doctor Sandler is already here. Dee's also down in Betty's room."

Dee was holding Betty in the sitting position, and Jerry had been listening to her chest. Jerry straightened up and shook his head. "I don't see anything, feel anything, or hear anything. She's got a low-grade fever this morning. Not a spike. She's alert, but I've decided to do another blood culture and catheterize her for a urine culture."

He stopped, raised his eyebrows, and looked down at Betty. "God, I hate to put her through all that, but she's still not waving."

"I'll get Morgan to help," Dee said.

"I'll help. Morgan and Brigid were busy getting ready for the morning's IV infusions of POMP," I said.

In the treatment room, Dee opened and prepared the IV tray. Jerry put on his gloves. I sat at the head of the surgical table, put one hand on the side of Betty's face, and placed my other hand on her left arm, which had the IV. While Jerry looked for a vein in the right arm, Dee moved to Betty's left side. Both Dee and I were ready to hold Betty down if necessary.

Betty grimaced when the needle went into her arm but didn't cry or scream. The same occurred when she was catheterized. Betty's steady gaze into my eyes was woeful. "Why are you doing this to me?' she seemed to ask.

When it was all over, I experienced a sensation of emptiness that must have been apparent in my posture, or perhaps on my face. I don't know how to describe the emotion. I really felt helpless, and this little girl—this tough, gentle little girl—went through all this without crying.

Jerry put his hand on my shoulder, "I know, Ben," he said. "I'd rather have them cry, kick, or scream. I hate sticking Betty more than any other patient."

• • •

By half past nine in the morning, 2 East was quiet. Betty was semi-comatose. There was extra traffic in and out of Betty's room. Not just the nurses and Jerry but also other mothers were visiting Betty. A nine-year-old patient of Rick's would slowly walk by Betty's door and try to peek in. The walls in the hall appeared darker, more gray than green.

Sally was receiving her POMP infusion. I stopped by her room to find Sally and Morgan looking at a book. Morgan looked up and explained that Mrs. Carter and one of the other mothers had taken Mrs. Miller to the cafeteria for a cup of coffee.

"Betty's sick," Sally said, looking at us as if we didn't know.

Sally knew. Everybody knew.

• • •

Rick and I were looking at the Board when Jerry came to see us at 3:20 p.m. "I need you to look at something," he said. "Betty has little lesions all over her body, and they're different from petechiae."

After washing hands, Jerry touched Betty on the shoulder and told her we were just going look at her skin. The lesions were small, like the head of a pin. Some were tan, others reddish, most somewhere in between.

Rick lightly ran the tips of his fingers over a few lesions and said, "Uh, you'd better feel these; most are slightly raised. Petechial eruptions are flat." Betty's mom was now standing with us at the bedside. Rick motioned me to the hall with his head.

"I'll be right back to explain the problem, Mrs. Miller," Jerry said.

"Jerry, those are septic emboli, probably caused by staph," Rick said when we were out in the hall.

"Oh…" Jerry said in a soft, falling voice. "That's what I was afraid they were. Are they going to turn into little abscesses?"

Rick shook his head. "It takes white blood cells to make pus. These are clumps of bacteria caught in the capillary bed of the skin; the clumps continued to grow, and the red color comes from small hemorrhages when the expanding bacterial mass breaks the capillary wall."

The three of us fell silent. This was the first case on the floor. We all knew it was a possible consequence of a low white count. We all had been looking at the skin of our patients hoping not to find it.

You can read about these types of things, hoping you'll be prepared for the future. You can forget what you have read, but when you come face-to-face with a problem, what you have experienced becomes indelible.

That Thursday night at the fence, I objectively mulled over the day. I wondered what was going to happen to Betty. Sadness crept in.

• • •

Friday. At 10:27 a.m., Betty died.

• • •

It happened again, like when Jennifer Johnson had progression of that facial swelling; staphylococcal infection of her lips spread down into her neck. For a day or two, there was no humor, no trivial remarks. Rick's patient, Jennifer, became my patient, Jerry's patient.

And now Betty Miller. Jerry, Rick, and I had talked about Betty early in the week. But when Betty developed staph sepsis, the three of us supported each other in silence. When Jennifer died, I didn't have to tell Rick I was sorry. He knew. Now Betty was gone, and it wasn't necessary to tell Jerry that I was going to miss her. It was as if anything said would be trivial.

Betty's postmortem exam resulted in a written report. No postmortem discussion of emotions occurred on 2 East.

• • •

The drive from NIH to home was a passage from the trauma of 2 East to the tranquility of Kirkhill. Key to this transition was the stretch of a two-lane road from Rockville to Darnestown.

From Rockville to Quince Orchard, there were several bends in Route 28. Not tight curves but enough to practice braking and downshifting my Austin-Healey, to come out of a curve with optimal power for a smooth transition to the next stretch of road, to listen to the motor purr or growl depending on the rpm. It wasn't speed I was after but the challenge of proper timing for optimal r.p.m. When well done, the motor, the gears, the tires, and I were one with the road.

A piece of road to induce peace of mind before carrot time at the fence.

Third Week

Monday, 9:00 a.m. Billy and I played with Bear. In the treatment room, at 9:35 a.m., I arranged the microscopic slides and the test tube containing an anticoagulant in preparation for his bone-marrow aspiration.

Morgan brought Billy into the room. He was crying, holding her hand. He didn't require two nurses to hold him down. He cried as his skin was cleansed. To make sure he didn't move too much during the aspiration, Morgan held his hips as the marrow was sucked out of his pelvis. Billy then stopped screaming, accepting Morgan's affectionate touch and her verbal assurance that it was all over.

For the first time, I added an additional routine to the bone-marrow aspiration. I asked Billy if I could carry him back to his room and his mother.

He put his arms up.

I carried Billy down the hall. Tears streamed down his cheeks, head on my shoulder.

It became my routine. I did it with all the toddlers and a few of the six- and seven-year-old patients.

There was something about those wet shoulders that made theoretical research and molecular biology seem irrelevant.

• • •

M onday at 11:10 a.m., a new patient, Robert Thurman, was listed for me on the Board.

Dee saw me in the hall and said, "Mr. and Mrs. Thurman are both here with Robert." She noted my surprised look. "It's unusual to have a father on the floor."

Robert was on his back, pale and covered with petechiae. He wore horn-rimmed glasses that partly obstructed a frown. After saying a few words to Robert, I introduced myself to his mother and father. Mr. Thurman handed me an envelope containing some laboratory data and a handwritten note from Robert's pediatrician in Alexandria.

"We were told that there are leukemia cells in Robert's blood and that he is anemic and has a low platelet count," Mr. Thurman said.

Before going into the grim details of the bone-marrow aspiration, I asked, "Does he prefer Bob or Bobby?"

"It's always Robert," his mother said. "His preference. He's quiet now, but he'll be full of questions about everything when he feels better." She smiled and put an arm around her son's shoulder.

A brief medical history and physical findings proved typical of the onset of leukemia. "I'll be in and out of the room most of the day and go into the details one step at a time."

After the marrow, I took the various vials of blood to the nurses' station and told Brigid I wanted the platelets from the blood bank stat; the blood transfusion would be a second priority, and the IV fluids should start at a modest rate.

When I returned from pathology, I told the parents, "The diagnosis is just as your pediatrician expected. It's our policy to tell the patient the name of his or her disease."

"We have already told Robert a little about leukemia; he knows the word," his father said.

I had just finished a medical history when Morgan came in with the platelets. Robert watched her connect IV tubing to a small plastic bag containing an opaque tan-colored suspension. "Robert," I said, "your parents tell me you are very curious and like to learn new words." He smiled for the first time. So I explained, in terms I hoped a nine-year-old would understand, "Platelets are very small packages of molecules that stop bleeding. These little red spots are points of bleeding into your skin. They're called petechiae. They occur when there aren't enough platelets in your blood." I had his full attention.

"What's a platelet look like?" Robert asked.

On a sheet of paper, I drew a three-inch smooth circle and a quarter-inch irregular circle. "If this big circle is a red blood cell, then this is a platelet," I said, pointing to the little circle.

Robert opened his mouth, but before he could ask his next question, his father suggested, "Son, let's try to remember the new words you've just learned. We can learn more tomorrow."

I had the feeling that Blood Cell Morphology 101 would not suffice in the long run, and I made a mental note to take Robert up to the pathology laboratory so we could both look down a double-headed microscope.

I was interrupted in writing my admitting note on Robert when Brigid handed me his blood counts and chemistries. His hemoglobin was about a third of normal. "Brigid, please call the blood bank. Tell 'em we want that unit of blood I ordered to be divided in half. I'll write a new order. We'll give him half today and half tomorrow so as not to overload his blood volume."

At 2:10 p.m., I explained to the parents, "We can't give Robert too much blood today. Only a small bag of blood will be hung this afternoon. More blood tomorrow."

During the course of our conversation, Mrs. Thurman said, "The president of our bridge club is going to organize a blood drive."

After expressing my gratitude on behalf of the blood bank, I thought, these are sophisticated people.

Back at my desk at 3:20 p.m., I looked at the blood chemistries before ordering POMP. Robert's uric acid was elevated, and there was a slight acidosis. Both conditions cause uric acid to crystallize in the kidney. I had already seen one patient with uric-acid nephropathy in Baby Boy Williams and didn't ever want to see another case.

It was now a quarter past four, and half a unit of blood was running. I listened to Robert's chest. His heart rate, though still rapid from the anemia, was slightly slower, suggesting we were administering fluids and blood products at a reasonable rate. I commented that the antileukemia drugs would be started tomorrow.

"Not tonight?" Mrs. Thurman asked.

Recognizing her disappointment, I said, "I'll be glad to explain the problem." Keep it simple, Humphrey, I thought. Uric-acid nephropathy is a complex problem. Then Tom Frei's discussion of the building blocks of DNA came back to me. Just reverse the process, I thought. "Robert's body is full of leukemia cells in his blood, bone marrow, enlarged spleen, and liver. The antileukemia drugs quickly kill leukemia cells. This results in lots of dead-cell debris, meaning proteins and DNA are dumped into the bloodstream. The body can break down the proteins into the original building blocks called amino acids and reutilize these to make new proteins for new healthy cells. But the body can't reutilize the old building blocks of DNA. These are changed into nonuseful molecules, one of which is uric acid."

Dad was taking notes. "OK."

"Too much uric acid in the blood blocks the kidneys' ability to make urine. Robert's uric acid is already high but not dangerously high. His kidneys are working fine, but if there were a rapid production of uric acid from killed leukemic cells, his kidneys would stop working."

Both Thurmans nodded.

"Robert is a little dehydrated. Sick patients tend not to eat or drink. He's not making a lot of urine—thus the increase in uric acid. The IV fluids he's receiving will correct the dehydration, and by tomorrow he should be making a lot of urine, enough to wash the acid out of his body. It will be safe to start killing leukemia tomorrow or the day after."

"I get it," Dad said, eliciting an audible sigh of relief from Mom.

A quarter to five, and I needed a break, so I took a copy of the POMP protocol out to my bench. After double-checking everything, I looked up to see my friend Squirrel. "Sorry, ol' buddy, I'm out of food; in fact, I'm sort of out of everything."

There wasn't anybody in the cafeteria I knew to join for dinner, so I ate alone, which this evening I preferred.

"Your puppy looks pretty good," Barbara said. "Why don't you go home?"

"I'll just pay a social call. Robert's interesting. Likeable. I'll tell his parents everything is set up for the night and that you'll call me if there's any change." Then with a smile and twinkle in my eye, I added, "If that's OK, Barbara."

"Oh, go on. You! You and Doctor Lottsfeldt and Doctor Sandler. You're all alike."

Back in the room, Mrs. Thurman said, "I've a confession to make. I thought the reason the drugs couldn't be started was because the pharmacy was closed. My husband and I were prepared to pay to have a pharmacist come back in to prepare the medicines for Robert."

"The pharmacy, blood bank, and key clinical laboratories are open and running twenty-four hours every day, including the weekends," I said.

"Thanks. And thanks for your explanations. It wasn't a matter of not trusting your judgment," Mr. Thurman said.

"No, no, no," I said. "Many parents want to know why this or that is done. It's useful for coping."

Walking down the hall to leave, I started to chuckle. Close the pharmacy now and then for a day or two, I thought. Delaying the delivery of POMP to the floor would have to save lives. Newspaper headlines: "Clinical Associate Decreases Death Rate at NCI." A lead article by me in

JAMA. I was tired and emotionally drained, laughing when I passed the nurses' station.

Barbara came out. "What's so funny, Doctor Humphrey?"

"I'm OK; just take good care of my little puppy Robert."

●　●　●

Tuesday nine o'clock. "Tell me about Thurman, Ben," Friereich said as he shuffled through my charts to find Robert's.

I presented the case, concluding with current lab and physical findings.

"You delayed starting POMP, Doctor Humphrey," Freireich said, looking at the orders.

I wanted to say it was because the pharmacy was closed but instead played it straight. "Robert's uric acid was elevated, he was slightly dehydrated, and his chemistries documented mild metabolic acidosis."

"Well. OK, that's right," he said, turning to Rick.

Well. OK. I didn't know Freireich even knew these words.

Later on my rounds, Robert looked great. He smiled and told me he was better. There were now a number of books on his bed. He was covered with petechiae, but there were no new lesions. He was anemic, but his heart rate was slower than last night. His liver and spleen were the same. "Robert, over here under your ribs on the left side is your spleen. It's bigger than normal because it too is full of leukemia cells."

"Mom, write those words down," Robert said, looking at his mother. Then he added, "Please."

I explained the orders of the day. "A blood transfusion to make you stronger, more fluid from your IV to wash out bad stuff from your blood, a light lunch, discuss the drugs we're going to give you to get rid of the leukemia cells, and then we'll start the drugs tomorrow. I want to check your uric-acid level one more time."

Later, I walked into Robert's room with my well-worn copy and two fresh copies of the POMP protocol. Mrs. Thurman thanked me and then to my surprise said, "We can read this tonight. Robert has an important question."

Robert beamed as the three adults turned their undivided attention to him. He could handle center stage. "I like books as much as soccer. I have my own dictionary and marked off words that I've looked up. I even know some words that aren't in my dictionary."

No longer uptight about having to explain all of chemotherapy, I chuckled despite myself and said, "I hope they're nice words, Robert."

His mother smiled. "I'm sure he knows some of those words too."

"What's your question, Robert?"

"What's going to happen to me?"

Dad's mood darkened, a frown replaced his smile, and his voice dropped. "Last year, we found a used set of *The World Book Encyclopedia* for Robert. Yesterday, he'd asked for the *L* volume, which we brought in and read to Robert. We all talked about the short article on leukemia. If Robert asks about something, we tell the truth as best we can; we don't hide things from him." His father handed me the *L* volume open to leukemia:

LEUKEMIA, lyoo, KE mih ah, is a fatal disease which affects the blood cells and the organs which produce them. Leukemia causes a great increase in the number of white blood cells, leukocytes, and a drop in the number of red blood cells... There is no useful treatment for severe cases of leukemia... See also Blood.

Opening the book to the front page, I read out loud, "Copyright 1955."

Dad had a tablet of yellow paper ready.

"Please write this down, Mr. Thurman," I said. "This article is out of date, and the statement 'There is no useful treatment for severe cases of leukemia' is not true."

"Robert," I said, "there is useful treatment for leukemia. Sixteen years ago—that's a looong time ago—a doctor named Farber gave children your age who had leukemia an antivitamin, and guess what?" I paused. "When the doctors did a bone-marrow aspirate a month later, they couldn't find *any* leukemia cells. That's called a remission."

Robert raised his eyebrows.

"One month from now, I'll have to do another bone-marrow aspiration. I don't expect to find any leukemia cells, which are sometimes called lymphoblasts or just plain blasts."

"That's very good news," his father said.

"Now, since Doctor Farber developed that first antileukemic drug, three more new and different drugs have been found that also cause remissions. Robert, you're going to get all four."

Mrs. Thurman kissed him on the forehead, as tears streamed down her cheeks.

"I need to check on Robert's lab test from this morning."

Mom's reaction was almost enough to make me cry. Robert was their only child.

Outside on my bench with a bag of peanuts, I consulted my impatient buddy Squirrel. "Another big question," I said with a sigh. "Last month Jimmy Paul wanted to know how children get into heaven, and now Robert wants to know what's going to happen to him."

By half past two, I was back. I repeated my explanation of the concept of remission, saying the treatment was tough and difficult. He'd lose his hair over the next month, and during the next five days, he'd be sick to his stomach.

There was one other item I ought to cover: relapses. How explicit was I going to be? I didn't know, so I just started an ad-lib monologue. "The problem today is not getting patients into remission. Not getting rid of the leukemia. The problem at present is that the leukemia can come back. That's called a relapse and can occur in several months or in a year or more. The current four-drug therapy, called POMP, is designed to try to prevent these relapses."

Robert had only one question. "Does the bald-headed kid I saw in the hall have leukemia?"

"Every patient on the floor is being treated for leukemia, Robert."

All the adults in the room were suffering from overload, so Robert and I chattered about movies he liked and his collection and love of books.

• • •

While I fed the horses their evening carrots, I reflected on Robert's question: "What's going to happen to me?" It was simple to look at the date of the encyclopedia and say leukemia was now a treatable disease. But what about long-term? The Thurmans were intelligent parents, information seekers. What would be a responsible answer to a question about whether any patients were being cured?

Earlier this month, I had seen a long-term survivor, Carl Shively. I knew Freireich had a few others like him in follow-up. Would it be fair to present this information to the Thurmans? Would that be too optimistic?

I wasn't used to thinking in this way, and I had that empty feeling in my gut. I was used to telling my adult patients about prognosis—being objective about what I said. But now, discussing the outcome of a presumed-fatal disease was associated with a responsibility. It would only be fair to say, "This is new therapy, and it's too early to know what the results will be."

• • •

During early-morning rounds, Mrs. Thurman explained, "For the rest of the week, I'll be with Robert in the mornings, and his dad will be with him in the afternoons. This arrangement has been approved by our respective firms. This way we both can get in six to eight hours of work."

On Monday and Tuesday, when both parents were on 2 East, each had a difference focus. Mr. Thurman was interested in the "whys" of treatment, while Mrs. Thurman was more interested in "What does this mean for Robert?"

When Mrs. Thurman asked me about preventing infection, I thought she might have talked to Mrs. Sullivan. "It's an important question. You may hear about some problems from other mothers also."

"I've learned about sepsis from Kathryn Sullivan. Her stories are far more vivid than the discussion of infection in the POMP protocol."

We discussed simple preventative measures, like handwashing and keeping Robert away from people who were sick.

We also talked about the bacteria that caused the infections; these germs generally came from the patient's own skin or bowel.

Mrs. Thurman then added, "Bacteria can also come from the mouth and infect the lips and neck."

God, I thought, she knows about Jennifer Johnson.

"When Robert goes back to school in September, should we keep him out for a few days in between courses of POMP when his white count is the lowest?"

"That's a good question. Not that I am aware of, but I'll ask Doctor Freireich."

"Who's Doctor Freewrite?" Robert asked, wanting to be in on the conversation.

I moved to the edge of Robert's bed. We practiced pronouncing *Freireich*. "He's my boss. Doctor Freireich's interested in the type of leukemia you have, Robert."

When I explained that Doctor Freireich was a world-famous physician, Robert said, "Gosh."

Holding up Robert's chart, I explained, "Yesterday, Doctor Freireich personally read your record, Robert."

Out came another "Gosh."

"Doctor Freireich works right here in this building,"

"Gosh."

"Yesterday, he asked me about you."

After four goshes, I decided to stop. "The other two doctors here on 2 East, Doctor Sandler and Doctor Lottsfeldt, also work for Doctor Freireich."

"You're lucky to work for a famous man," a wide-eyed Robert said.

I lied and said yes.

Lucky wasn't the word we were likely to use to describe our relationship with Emil J. Freireich, MD. We were supposed to call him Jay but after his first lecture; Jerry had dubbed him *schmuck*, and the title stuck.

• • •

In his office, I asked Jay, "Do kids need to be taken out of school at any time because of low counts?"

"No." He continued to pore over a chart.

"Mrs. Thurman wanted to know. Remember, she's the one that organized a blood drive. Robert Thurman's a very inquisitive nine-year-old. I've told Robert about your research and that you're world-famous."

Without looking up from his work, he said, "I'm not sure that's true."

"Robert's never met anyone who is famous. He just wants to shake your hand."

Jay looked up, put his pencil down, and smiled. "I'll be glad to do that." He leaned back in his chair. "The first three years I was here, I did it all. There were no clinical associates. I liked talking to the kids and their moms. I think you guys have the better part of the work that has to be done around here."

I thought to myself, I'm not sure that's true.

On our way to Robert's room, I told him about his love of books and soccer and a bit about the parents.

As Freireich walked into Robert's room, a metamorphosis occurred. A broad smile swept across Jay's face. "Good afternoon, Mrs. Thurman, I'm Doctor Freireich. I want to thank you for the blood drive you organized." He washed his hands and went over to Robert. "I'm pleased to see books on your bed. Let me feel your tummy, young man."

I was amazed at this performance, but it wasn't a show.

"Yes, the spleen is definitely smaller than what you noted at diagnosis," he said to me. Smiling at Mrs. Thurman he added, "That's good. That's great!"

"Gosh, you're famous," Robert said no longer able to contain himself.

Then to my astonishment, Jay paused, lay his hand on Robert's shoulder and said, "Well, I don't know about that, but I have been doing clinical research on leukemia here at NIH for a number of years," then he added, "Here in America. You need to ask Doctor Humphrey about his research. He's worked not only in America but also in Europe."

"Gosh."

After a couple of "Nice to meet yous," I followed Freireich out into the hall. My mouth wasn't hanging open, but I must have looked surprised.

"You're surprised I knew about your research," he said in a neutral tone.

"Well, ah, yes sir. I appreciate your seeing Robert and his mom." I remembered how he had handled Rick when Jennifer was dying of mucositis and added, "Tact has not been your strongest suit, Doctor Freireich." A dumb thing to say, but all of my decorum was gone for the moment.

Still reflective he told me, "Eighteen months ago you and a lot of other guys applied for an appointment to this service. Out of that pile, I selected approximately ten applications, re-read 'em and even called the individuals you listed as references before selecting you, Lottsfeldt, and Sandler."

I took a deep breath and swallowed.

Looking me in the eye with a smile of self-satisfaction, he said, "And here's the reason I know so much about you and the other associates.

You only have to deal with one individual, me. I have to deal with all three of you. It's three against one, and I always win."

• • •

Three piles of hay over the fence, make sure the water tank was full, enjoy a few moments watching Domino wolf down his hay – these were part of my morning respite on any day of the week. On most Saturday and Sunday mornings, this reprieve lasted longer.

Being on call, I had already phoned 2 East to check on Robert. Barbara told me, "Your puppy's fine. You don't have to rush in. Take it easy this morning."

Robert greeted me at 9:35 a.m. with, "I've been working on four new words."

"What are they?"

"*Platelet, petechiae, ero – e- rith-row – erythrocyte,* and *leukemia,*" Robert grinned. "Dad helped me last night, Mom this morning. I know that erythrocyte is another name for a red blood cell, but I like the bigger word."

I chuckled. "You never know when you're going to need to be able to say *erythrocyte.* Next time you order a hamburger, tell the waiter you want one without erythrocytes."

Mrs. Thurman and I helped Robert use his new words in simple sentences. His mother smiled when Robert said, "My leukemia is being treated. Dad and I talked about that last night." He paused. Then in a lower tone, he said to me, "Mom and I talked about that this morning."

"Robert knows this is a serious disease," Mrs. Thurman said. "I've learned a lot from Kathryn Sullivan. I know about Billy and Bear. Fever and sepsis. I also know about Betty Miller. It's important for me to spend time with Kathryn. Billy is her only child. It's like having a soul mate."

The room was quiet.

"Kathryn Sullivan and Helen Miller have experienced things I didn't know existed." She shook her head as if to break the mood. "I understand you're training a horse, Doctor Humphrey."

• • •

Robert completed the last dose of POMP on Saturday. Because of anemia, he'd not been discharged but had received a blood transfusion on Sunday. The nurses had gone over some of the precautions for patient care after remission-induction therapy: fever, nosebleeds, and so on.

Earlier, Mrs. Thurman had asked me about soccer, not in front of Robert but in the hall. While soccer is not supposed to be a contact sport, we discussed the trauma that can occur. She wasn't surprised that soccer wasn't a good idea; Kathryn Sullivan had told her about Billy's bloody noses. I suggested she and her husband try to think of some new activity for Robert.

Discharge instructions were generally a happy time for me but not today. Mom and Dad were both in the room. "No soccer, Robert," I said. Robert might be a bookworm, but he loved soccer. "I'm sorry."

He slumped over in bed.

When I asked, Robert told me about one of his new words, *platelets*. "What do platelets do, Robert?"

"They stop bleeding."

Reviewing the fact that during the next couple of weeks, he might not have enough platelets to stop bleeding if he hurt himself, I said, "You might have to come back to the hospital for a platelet transfusion. So, no soccer, no roughhousing, stay off your bike, and for the next month be careful."

Robert's mom put her arm around her son and said, "We'll think of other things to do."

Walking out of the room, I felt crummy.

Mr. Thurman caught up with me. "Doctor Humphrey, Robert's been asking for a dog for over a year. It might be a good time to give in. Is there any problem with a child receiving chemotherapy having a dog?"

"Not that I've read, Mr. Thurman but I know someone to ask. We have a pediatrician on the staff," I said and then added, "He's also an oncologist." I called Rick at home, and he knew of no reason why Robert couldn't have a puppy.

In fifteen minutes, I was back. "Mr. Thurman, Doctor Lottsfeldt, that pediatrician I spoke of, says it's OK."

Dad went over to his son. "Why don't we go out and look for a puppy when we get home?"

"Gosh," Robert howled. He jumped out of bed and gave his dad a hug. My little ex–soccer player asked if they could buy a book on dogs on the way home.

• • •

Back at Kirkhill in the early evening, I went to the fence. A warm breeze, and the aroma of woodsmoke from a farmer burning logs from some land-clearing project. I was glad that I didn't have to ponder my day or week in the dark. What a week it had been. The incident with the encyclopedia reminded me of Alexander Pope: "A little learning is a dangerous thing."

The patient education of the Thurmans had been exhausting but also rewarding. I never had that experience dealing with adults. I had done it all by myself and not as a member of a medical team. "Exhausting but also rewarding." It was as if I had done something important.

For the first time in my professional life, I felt like I had been a physician.

Fourth Week

Monday. Three names on the Board: Tammy Long, Michelle Karr, and Todd Yardley. All were refreshing in their differences: Tammy, the quiet preadolescent who wanted to look pretty; Michelle, the snuggle bunny for my lap; and Todd, the boy with a dog named Ralph. Three mothers, each with different coping styles, all easy to respect. All three patients were symptom-free: no bleeding, fevers, or bone pain. Three brief examinations were normal: no signs of petechiae, splenomegaly, or lymphadenopathy. It was a good morning until a quarter past ten when I had to begin the breaking of bones.

By a quarter to noon, I knew that all three were in remission.

Telling a mother that her son or daughter was still in remission was both a relief and a pleasure.

• • •

After lunch and before starting the IVs and chemotherapy, I had time for a social call.

Sitting up in her bed, Tammy wore her auburn wig, makeup, her pretty floral nightgown, and a smile. Even an internist could tell that Tammy and her mother had gone to some trouble to put this all together. She was a pied beauty. Good nickname. Tonight, I'd reread Gerard Manley Hopkins to double-check on the meaning of "Pied Beauty."

"Wow, Tammy. You look like you're sixteen." It must have been the right thing to say. Tammy turned and lowered her head. I put a finger under her chin, turned her head up, and made some admiring remarks about the eyeliner, the rouge, the color of her lipstick, and the perfume she wore. The scent was floral, and Tammy wore a lot of it.

"Tammy has an older sister, fourteen, who's learning to wear makeup. On special occasions Tammy's allowed to wear makeup, which I apply. She'd overdo it if I let her do it all."

"Tammy, you're beautiful," I said.

"We went to J. C. Penney. Tammy picked out the nightgown herself. We'll take it off and wear a hospital gown when the drugs start," Mrs. Long said. "She also chose the perfume; I'm afraid she's wearing a little too much."

Mrs. Long had created a great distraction. It was as if the three of us were pretending we weren't on 2 East.

• • •

When I walked into Todd's room, he exploded with, "What kind of dog does Dracula have?"

Not wanting to spoil his riddle, I said, "A Transylvanian terrier?"

"Nooo," Todd said with delight. "A bloodhound! Do ya get it?"

Mrs. Yardley reminded me of my joke in July about the average height of all dogs being something over four feet. She explained that Todd wanted to have his own joke for me, so they went to the library and found a children's book on dog jokes, riddles, and stories. "Watch out, Doctor Humphrey, he's loaded with riddles." Then turning to Todd, she said, "It's Monday, and Doctor Humphrey is very busy. Save your riddles for the rest of the week."

"It'll be at least an hour before the pharmacy will have the infusions ready. I can't think of anything more important to do than talk about dogs." I told Todd about Shonto, the water trough, and Domino, promising to bring in a picture.

"How can you tell if you have a dumb dog?" Ralph asked. Before I could answer, he interrupted with, "It chases parked cars!"

How could one not smile? Mrs. Yardley was pleased at her son's performance. I was lost in Todd's world. The internist was gone from the room.

"Todd, here's a line from a poem for you," I said. "A door is what a dog is always on the wrong side of."

107

Mrs. Yardley smiled and said, "Ogden Nash." She asked if I liked poetry and why I was smiling.

"Todd takes me back to my youth," I said. "It's a pleasant trip."

• • •

Ending this round of social calls, I found Michelle sitting in her mother's lap.

Mrs. Karr held out her daughter so I could take Michelle. We had a prolonged conversation.

"The last time before 2 East that I remember having a baby in my lap was when I was six. The baby was my sister, and my dad took our picture."

Mrs. Karr possessed a great deal of insight. She asked probing questions and kept the conversation going. She knew I wanted to keep her snuggle bunny in my lap. But I also think she enjoyed watching other people take pleasure in holding her child. I had noted that when she handed Michelle to a nurse, a smile of pride came over her face. This sharing of Michelle made everybody happy.

• • •

Every now and then, the clinical associates, as we preferred to think of ourselves, would receive a memo from the military side of the US Public Health Service. These memos used our military rank, lieutenant commander. One from this series informed us we were welcome to dine at the officers' club at the Bethesda Naval Hospital. In addition, if we were sick or injured, we were to report to the triage office, and we could shop at the PX. The latest epistle was an order: "Report on 26 August at 1500 to the classroom adjacent to 12 East for a briefing on your responsibilities as officer of the day."

At precisely 3:00 p.m., an officer and a member of the shore patrol marched into the room. The officer, his hat smartly tucked under an arm, was a full commander and his bearing that of a lifelong professional in the navy. Uniform impeccable, he was as stiff as the starch in his shirt. I wasn't impressed with him, but his associate was a different matter. He was bearing a .45-caliber automatic and a nightstick.

"At ease," the officer said as a matter of habit. We were all sitting down.

He looked us over. I gathered he was used to dealing with clinical associates and our disregard for military protocol. Turning to the sailor, he said, "Roll call."

"Yes, sir." The sailor produced a list. "Commander Lottsfeldt?"

Rick raised his hand.

"We require a verbal response," the commander interjected. "'Here' or 'Present' will do." Rick complied, as did the rest of us until Mike, one the associates from 12 East, was called, and he loudly clicked his heels as he responded, which was ignored.

Commander Wallace introduced himself and stated he was responsible for security at both NIH and the Bethesda Naval Hospital. He explained that while we might think of the NIH campus as a hospital and a group of research buildings, it was in fact a military base, requiring one individual each day to serve as officer of the day. Each of us would serve one day in October. We would be required to sleep overnight on the base. Other information was passed out: locations of the on-call quarters, important telephone numbers, and so on. Then he made a mistake. "Are there any questions?"

"Do I get a six-shooter?" Mike asked. He received an icy stare. "Well, how about a crossbow?"

"That will be all, gentlemen," the commander said through gritted teeth and stormed out the door.

Mike continued, "Worst case of poker spine, or ankylosing spondylitis as we call it in medicine, I've ever seen.

"Well," I said, "if the Russians invade the place, you don't need a weapon. Give 'em a course of POMP. That'll stop 'em dead in their tracks."

• • •

The primary problem for the clinical associates on 2 East was chemotherapy-induced toxicity. Less common, but more tragic, was a relapse. That meant POMP was discontinued, and the patient was eligible for a new experimental drug, daunomycin.

By now, Jerry and I were accustomed to thinking of POMP as a phase III clinical trial and daunomycin as a phase II trial. When we first arrived on 2 East, Rick was kind enough to review the concept with Jerry and me. Rick made it simple. In phase I, a new drug is given to humans for the first time to determine a tolerable dose. In phase II, that same dose is given to patients with one specific cancer to determine efficacy. In our world, daunomycin was being tested in patients with ALL. Phase III tests which drug or combination of drugs will give the best result. On 2 East, the question was, would POMP be better than any other published combination of antileukemic agents?

We knew from Jay that daunomycin had caused, in some patients, a reduction in bone-marrow leukemia.

Tuesday-morning rounds with Jay. I presented each patient: all three were receiving the second day of therapy.

"Jerry, how are your patients doing?" Jay asked. Jerry presented two patients on POMP, both on schedule.

Rick handed a chart to Jay and explained his patient was on schedule.

"Where's Jason Saunder's chart? He relapsed yesterday," Jay asked.

"The parents didn't want to try any experimental drugs and only wanted to take Jason home," Rick said.

Jay frowned. "Dammit! No daunomycin! We need new and better drugs. That's a promising agent. In the future it might complement the agents of POMP and reduce relapses and drug resistance. Jimmy Paul,

Ben's patient, achieved a partial remission on daunomycin. Did you mention Jimmy when you were discussing experimental therapy with Jason's mom?"

"No, sir," Rick said. "I know the importance of phase II research, Jay."

"Your knowing that, Doctor Lottsfeldt, is all fine and well, but Jason wasn't registered on the daunomycin trial. A lost opportunity to help evaluate this agent. If the data hold up, daunomycin will be in the next frontline protocol."

• • •

I made my social rounds at 1:20 p.m. when the pharmacy would be delivering the infusion bags of chemotherapy.

Todd talked about Ralph. I shared a story from my boyhood about our family dog, Betsy, as well as family joke that I was seven before I realized one of my two sisters was a cocker spaniel. Todd frowned, and Mrs. Yardley laughed.

Tammy showed me a few pictures from a fashion magazine. To my surprise, Mrs. Long joined the two of us. That was my first real conversation with both mother and daughter.

Brigid was already in Michelle's room. The first bag of prednisolone was lying on the bedside table. Mrs. Karr was holding Michelle quietly on her lap, and Brigid was sitting next to her, leaning forward and holding Michelle's hand.

"I was sorry to hear about Jason Saunders," Mrs. Karr said. "He was a sweet little boy. Brigid and I were just talking about his relapse."

Bad news travels fast on 2 East.

"We all felt bad about Jason," Brigid said.

I had that sinking feeling. What will I say to you, I thought, when Michelle relapses?

• • •

A good coffee break was about to get better.

"Jerry, the other day I saw Morgan coming out of one of the rooms wearing a broad smile," I said. "When I asked what was up, she said, 'Doctor S. is in there tellin' tall tales about Maine fog to his patient, Jonathan. Get him to tell you the story.' Jerry, I didn't know you were from Maine."

"Ayuh, I'm a native Maine'ah. You betcher life," Jerry said in what I assumed was a Down East accent. "We've got real fogs. Not those little pea-soupers off Lake Michigan that creep in on little kitten feet but fogs off Casco Bay that prowl in on big panther paws. Fogs so thick you can drive a spike in 'em if you've got a thick hammer and you can hang a heavy coat on that there spike."

On and on Jerry went, and Rick and I were in stitches—two six-foot-tall five-year-olds.

• • •

On 2 East, there were two basic threats: a bone-marrow relapse, which meant death, and chemotherapy-induced toxicity, which could mean death.

Mrs. Yardley lived with both. She was intelligent and well-read, and I liked the fact that she knew Ogden Nash. That fit with her sense of humor. She had a nice way with words. For example, she didn't say that Todd's dog was named after an imaginary friend but rather that there had been "a transmigration of a soul." But she could be pragmatic and honest in dealing with her son's cancer: "The bone-marrow aspiration and the start of five days of chemotherapy are a vivid reminder that Todd is not cured," Mrs. Yardley had said in July.

She was proud of her son. And why not? Once the ice was broken, Todd was full of life and humor and wanted to participate in the social aspects of our relationship. After the humor we shared last month on dogs, it was Todd who got a book of dog jokes. He wasn't going to give me an edge on comedy, and he kept me on my toes.

On Thursday afternoon, Todd spiked a fever. Morgan told me in the nurses' station. I was angry at the news—the same type of anger Freireich exhibited when he acknowledged Jason Saunders had relapsed. After I calmed down, I went to Todd's room.

Mrs. Yardley already knew about the fever.

I reviewed the procedure. "Blood culture, IV antibiotics. If no bacteria are found in the blood and there's no fever for two days, we'll discontinue the IV antibiotics, and Todd can go home. If bacteria are found in the blood, then ten days of IV antibiotics."

"I know, Doctor Humphrey." She paused. "But it is important to me to hear it again from you."

On Saturday, I would stop Todd's IV antibiotics, because there was an increase in his white count. On Sunday, he was discharged to go home and see Ralph. Possible sepsis was a short-term threat that had not materialized.

• • •

That Thursday night at the fence, I was in a bad mood. I never swore out loud, but tonight I thought, fuck objectivity, fuck POMP, fuck toxicity…I wasn't ordinarily prone to anger, and one event would almost never cause the rage I felt tonight. It was time that had gotten to me. Time on 2 East! I was tired of writing orders that could cause toxicity, tired of looking for toxicity all week long, tired of finding toxicity, and tired of watching patients die of toxicity.

• • •

Friday morning, I told Rick and Jerry about Todd's fever. For once I revealed how I felt about my friend Todd: how he needed to go home to Ralph and how his mother was in limbo.

Jerry was concerned about a mouth sore in an afebrile seven-year-old.

Rick shrugged. "None of mine are sick or toxic; one will be going home today and the other on Saturday."

Jerry asked, "How is it you've got a patient getting POMP over the weekend?"

"Rick, you're not having the toxicity that Jerry and I are seeing in our patients. It's got to be something other than experience. Yes, POMP is toxic. We all know that, but it's not as toxic in your hands," I said.

I could see that Rick was working through something. Jerry started to talk, but Rick motioned with a wave of his hand and shake of his head for Jerry to be quiet.

"Uh, OK," he said. "It has to do with the peripheral blood count. If a patient is anemic, I give POMP on Monday, because you can always give a blood transfusion. The same thing with a low platelet count. But a low white count is different. Only time and marrow recovery will correct a low white count." He sat up. "That's it," he said. "I guess I use the criteria we used in Minnesota for starting or stopping chemotherapy. If I'm worried that POMP will wipe out white-cell recovery, I delay therapy, even if only for a day or two."

"How do you delay starting the drugs?" Jerry asked. "We're supposed to start POMP on Monday."

"It's simple. I do what I can to allow the bone marrow to recover," Rick said. "On Tuesday morning before rounds, I order a chest x-ray or send the patient for some procedure in another clinic—dental or ENT. When the patient leaves 2 East, his or her chart goes along with the patient. When Freireich asks what's going on, I tell him I'm just checking something out but that everything is OK. Then the POMP is started on Tuesday afternoon or, on a couple of occasions, Wednesday." He paused. "Just a day or two can make a big difference."

"Can a day or two of deferring therapy really be that important?" I asked.

"I think so, Ben. A recovering marrow contains a lot of young white cells that need a day to mature and be released into the blood. They're dividing. Dividing cells are very sensitive to chemotherapy." He paused. "I think it helps. I'm a trained pediatric oncologist—gonna give drugs to kids the rest of my life. I just don't ever again want to see a Jennifer Johnson."

Jerry and I were quiet. Neither of us shouted, "That's it," or, "Great idea."

"Uh, you guys are welcome to use the same technique."

We sat together in silence. No one wanted to see another Jennifer Johnson, no one wanted to have to say good-bye to another Betty Miller, and no one wanted to be giving IV antibiotics over the weekend to a patient in remission, who might have sepsis, who might die. Just a day or two of delay might prevent some of this. The issue was obvious: the dilemma of needing to avoid severe toxicity versus protocol compliance.

We put our heads together. Rick had absolutely no problems with Jerry and me using this approach, but we couldn't have all the patients off the floor getting chest x-rays. Freireich wasn't stupid. He was bright, observant, and committed to the protocol. So we devised a plan. We'd meet every Monday morning before lunch and look at all the admissions for POMP. If possible, we'd give them all POMP and pray. If one or more patients were judged to be a risk for severe granulocytopenia, we'd get the one at greatest risk off the floor. It wasn't going to be a question of whose turn it was but which patient was at greatest risk.

• • •

August was over. None of my patients had relapsed, but it was just a matter of time. None had died of toxicity—again a question of time. The same old question came to me. What do I have to know to be a good physician for my little patients? What do I have to do to survive?

SEPTEMBER

First week

On this refreshingly cool Monday morning, the sun was sweeping away the dew from the meadow. A time to enjoy the tasks of distributing sweet feed and hay and filling the water trough. None of my patients were hospitalized, so no need to rush into NIH.

The Healey's top was down—lots of time for a slow drive into Bethesda. Normally, I drove in worrying about a patient, the top up to save time.

The first week in September meant the beginning of fall, my favorite time of the year. The school year started after Labor Day, and as a child I liked school. Red and yellow leaves raked into piles for jumping and then burning. Billowing clouds of dense white smoke were fun to run through, leaf smoke the aroma of autumn.

In the NIH parking lot, I put the top up and walked into the world of biomedical research and mothers and children dealing with leukemia.

• • •

I looked at the Board, the harbinger of my week ahead. There were two names listed for me: John Graham and Sarah Thompkins.

John, eleven, had responded to radiation therapy for his abdominal lymphoma but experienced severe nausea and vomiting with POMP. He was the most worrisome patient I was following since he had withdrawn after his first course of chemotherapy.

I smiled as I thought of Sarah. There's a challenge for you: this week, see if you can get this six-year-old to smile. There wasn't an obsequious bone in her body. She'd have her Barbie and would politely set her doll aside to allow me to examine her, but she never cracked a smiled.

• • •

"I admitted John Graham this morning, Doctor Humphrey," Brigid said. "I don't think Mrs. Graham's doing very well. She looks like she hasn't slept for days."

Already in his hospital gown, John held the top sheet close to his chest. I said hello to him but didn't go to his bedside.

Between the windowed wall and the hospital bed was a large padded armchair, which Mrs. Graham had pulled up to the head of the bed. She looked up at me, eyebrows raised, and I noted dark circles under her eyes. Sleep deprivation is a sign of depression.

I felt helpless, as if I'd never gone to medical school.

"The last few nights, I've slept better just knowing we'd be here," she said.

"I'm sorry there isn't more we can do for you and John."

"Oh, I want to show you something. We've been drawing. John has an eye for detail." Turning to her son, she asked, "John, is it OK if I show Doctor Humphrey your drawing of our house?"

John nodded once.

Mrs. Graham unfolded a large sheet of white paper. She explained, "The details are exactly like our home. The number and placement of the windows, the chimney, and the type of front door are accurate."

It was all there, a small black drawing, down in the lower-left-hand corner of the page. The rest was blank. A fence, drawn in heavy, bold lines, surrounded the house and isolated it.

"Is there a fence around your home, Mrs. Graham?"

She gazed at the drawing and sighed. "No."

I sighed and exchanged a glance with John's mother.

As I left his room, Brigid and Mrs. Thompkins were waiting in the hall.

"I'm gonna take Julia for a cup of coffee," Mrs. Thompkins said.

"Mrs. Thompkins, I'll see Sarah later. There's no rush; you take your time over coffee."

"I'll stay with John," Brigid said.

• • •

Sarah Thompkins wasn't glad to see me, but I couldn't complain about her behavior. When I examined her, she always cooperated and didn't require even one nurse to restrain her during a marrow aspiration or venipuncture.

"Good morning, Sarah."

To my surprise, she responded, "Good morning, Doctor." I couldn't remember if we had ever exchanged such a salutation.

Mrs. Thompkins volunteered all the important information about the last month.

"Thank you," I said when my physical exam was over.

Mrs. Thompkins nudged her daughter. "You tell your doctor, 'You're welcome.'" Sarah complied.

Out in the hall, I thought, Sarah had leukemia, and the prognosis wasn't good, but Mrs. Thompkins was still raising her daughter.

• • •

Later in the day, Mrs. Thompkins stopped me in the hall. "Doctor, I'm sorry Sarah don't talk much."

"Mrs. Thompkins, she doesn't require two nurses to hold her down for a bone-marrow aspiration or for starting an IV. That takes a *lot* of stress out of those procedures for both the nurses and me."

"I've told Sarah you don't like them needles; I've told her you like children. I know about the puzzles, talkin' about dogs—you know, that sort of thing."

"Mrs. Thompkins, a bone-marrow aspiration really hurts. Sarah has good reason not to like me, and that's OK—rational—understandable. Besides, Sarah greeted me today with a good morning."

"Well, that's just good manners. Her pa and I insist on that. She'd get slapped if she was sassy."

Indirectly I suggested that being "slapped" wasn't really a good idea when the platelet count was low. To end on a positive note, I pointed out that Sarah had an affectionate relationship with her and that was what was important.

"Yes, but…"

I put up both my hands with palms out. "Mrs. Thompkins, I like Sarah. I too was raised on good manners, but I was also taught to respect individuality. Please don't ask her to change or pretend she likes me."

● ● ●

Before I walked into the nurses' station, Dee informed me, "John's mom wants to see you."

Mrs. Graham had forgotten to tell me this morning the good news about John's school. "To be honest, Doctor Humphrey," she said, "when you walk into the room, my mind goes blank, especially on Monday mornings before you have the results of the bone-marrow test. I'm sort of in limbo, like the future is. Like the future's something to fear."

The remark sank in, but I'd deal with it later.

"We live in a small suburb of Alexandria, an upper-income community. Our taxes are high, but our schools are excellent. John's school has just hired a clinical psychologist, a Doctor White, and she seems very interested in John's case. We told her what we had tried. She's going to talk to John's teachers and asked us to make a list of his favorite subjects. She's also going to suggest that our son be excused from stressful subjects or activities."

"Great."

"Doctor White gave us her school and home telephone numbers. My husband will take time off from work for a weekly meeting, and she'll work with John, three times a week."

What Mrs. Graham said next made me sit back in my chair.

"Doctor Humphrey, I'll give you a progress report next month." Mrs. Graham paused. "Whatever we learn might be of value for some other child having the same problem."

• • •

Between the door marked 2 East and the one that opened into the floor was a waiting room, an open area. On the far wall, a long couch sat flanked by a series of armchairs. They were all covered with a smooth synthetic material. A bank of windows over the long couch offered natural light to this open space. You had to pass through the waiting room to enter or leave 2 East.

The nursing staff requested all mothers respect rest hour, from 1:00 p.m. to 2:00 p.m., so the younger patients could take a nap. As no one was hauled off to the treatment room, it was also the safest hour of the day for patients, their mothers, the nurses, and physicians. I don't recall any problems occurring during rest period. Even death took that hour off.

The nurses could do their charting and paperwork without interruption.

If we weren't busy, Rick would occasionally have lunch with his wife, Jody. I sometimes signed out and went for a long walk and generally spent time with my buddy Squirrel. Jerry often joined a friend for lunch in Georgetown.

But the mothers of 2 East were busy. Most of them gathered in the waiting room. As my personal paranoia about POMP and fear of treating pediatric patients abated, I became aware of the dynamics of the couch. At times, two or three mothers would sit close to one another, sometimes taking the hand of another holding a handkerchief. Here where one mother could relate to another, friendships would be forged, a network of support would be established, and mothers could cry freely.

• • •

The trees had started to turn; the temperature was mild and my mood mellow. Drinking coffee downstairs, the three of us were down in the dumps. It had been a rough week for Jerry. A five-year-old died on Monday. A two-year-old needed an IV restarted on Tuesday and again on Wednesday. On both days, Rick had had to stick the patient twice to establish a flowing IV after Jerry failed three times, and I hadn't been able to get a word out of John. I'd been of little value to his mother.

"It's September," Jerry said. "We've got over ten more months to go on 2 East." He looked at Rick. "Well, Ben and I, as internists, have ten more months of pediatric oncology to go."

It was time for some humor. I sang to Jerry, "'Try to remember the kind of September, when life was slow and oh, so mellow.'"

"Hey, I really like that, Ben," Rick said.

"It's not original; it's from *The Fantasticks*," I said.

Jerry chimed in, "'Try to remember when life was so tender, when dreams were kept beside your pillow.'"

I didn't know he was a romantic. It was a side of him we hadn't seen before.

Jerry said he knew all the words to "Try to Remember" and that *The Fantasticks* was a great date. "Really gets 'em in the mood, and there's that great line, 'Love was an ember about to billow.'"

I laughed out loud and pounded the table. "You're impossible, Jerry."

"Ben, you know, we ought to get Rick an LP of the music and words. He's gonna be a father: 'Plant a turnip, get a turnip, not a brussels sprout.'"

I had forgotten that song, but Jerry knew the words.

Rick went to the library; Jerry and I walked onto 2 East. After we cleared the door, Jerry stopped me. Like an actor without a mask in a Greek tragedy, Jerry said, "When I look down this hall, I'm reminded of another line from *The Fantasticks*:

'Try to remember when life was so tender, that no one wept except the willow.'"

My comrade in arms could look down this long dark hall and see more than gray-green paint. *The Fantasticks* sang to me the rest of that day and into the weekend.

Second Week

On Monday morning at a quarter past eight, I was greeted with, "Doctor Humpfee." Sally was holding up a new puzzle still in its cellophane wrapping. She was sitting on her bed in a hospital gown. Next to her was Pebbles. Bald-headed, wearing a smile, Sally was beautiful.

Sally started to tell me a story. Mrs. Carter in her cordial way gently interrupted her daughter. "Save that for tomorrow; it's Monday."

I told her it was a light morning and I wanted to hear about Betsy, Sally's friend.

Listening to one of Sally's verbal routines, I wondered if this three-year-old knew that as long as she talked and I listened, I wasn't going to hurt her. During the physical exam, the smile never left my face. As usual, she enchanted me.

At 9:25 a.m., I carried a sobbing Sally back to her room, put her down on her bed, and pulled the sheet over her legs and chest. She let me hold her hand while wiping the last of her tears away with the other.

At 10:10 a.m., it was determined there was no leukemia in the marrow. Sally greeted me. "Doctor Humpfee."

"We've been working on the proper pronunciation of your name, Doctor Humphrey," Mrs. Carter said.

"I've already acquired too many titles and labels. Sally's a charmer, and having been given a special name by your daughter is refreshing. To hear Sally cry out, 'Doctor Humpfee,' brightens my day."

Mrs. Carter smiled and nodded.

"I remember the first time I was called 'Doctor Humphrey.' Pretty neat, I thought. The novelty soon wore off, and the title, doctor, generally meant a demand was going to be placed on my time. Then, there was 'Herr Doktor' when I was in Germany and now 'commander' at the officers' club at Bethesda Naval Hospital."

"But Sally doesn't call you 'Doctor Humpfee' when we're at home. You're her 'puzzle doctor.'"

"Neat! Come here, Sally. That's great! You know, Sally, someday I hope to be a teacher at a medical school. Do you know what I'm going to have painted on my office door?"

She shook her head.

In a solemn tone, I said, "G. Bennett Humphrey, MD, PhD, SCPD."

Mrs. Carter kept the game going. "What does SCPD stand for?"

I turned to Sally. "SCPD stands for..." Tapping her four times lightly on the chest, I continued, "Sally—Carter's—Puzzle—Doctor."

Mrs. Carter laughed.

That night when I got back to Kirkhill, Shonto wagged her tail, and Domino and the Thoroughbreds nickered, pawing the ground. I liked these bucolic forms of address. It was a wonderful way to end the day, just as "Doctor Humpfee" had been a marvelous way to start it.

• • •

On the Board was Penny Tapley. My new patient. Walking into Penny's room, I started to introduce myself to a woman holding a stout two-year-old. Penny sat on that lap like a boulder. She had a square face, her full cheeks were pale, and her sandy-colored hair was pulled neatly into a pigtail. Penny wore a full-skirted dress decorated with faded blue and red teddy bears that looked like it had been washed a thousand times and worn by scores of little girls.

"I'm not Penny's mother, Doctor. I'm Virginia Jenkins, a volunteer from the county. Penny's mother can't get time off from work. Our church has a volunteer organization to help families in need, mostly home care or situations like this."

I pulled up a chair and sat down, now a habit when talking to mothers, to indicate I had time to spend and wasn't about to bolt out the door. My shoulders dropped as I thought of what we were going to put Penny through in the next few days: a bone-marrow aspirate, an IV, nauseating drugs, a strange place, and no Mom.

Mrs. Jenkins handed me an envelope containing three sheets of paper. On a prescription sheet was a handwritten note by a Doctor Bodey requesting a complete blood count from a laboratory. He had suspected leukemia because of Penny's pallor and his finding an enlarged liver and spleen. A laboratory sheet from a pathologist reported a low hemoglobin and the presence of circulating leukemia cells. Finally there was a typed letter from a social worker who had helped coordinate the admission to NIH and made the arrangements for a volunteer to accompany Penny to Bethesda.

Mrs. Jenkins looked like a grandmother, probably in her early fifties. She had short graying curly hair, was a bit stout, and presented a face that bore a few wrinkles. She did her best to answer my questions, made a few notes about missing information, and said she'd have that for me tomorrow.

The social history caused me to sigh. The father had abandoned the family before Penny was born. "Took the pickup truck, his guns, and his clothes," Mrs. Jenkins said, curling the left side of her upper lip, "and just snuck out of town. Good riddance, I say."

The rest of the family history was a bit more positive. There was an eight-year-old brother and a ten-year-old sister. Penny was cared for during school hours by neighbors and afterward by her siblings.

Mrs. Jenkins sensed my astonishment about Penny's mom having to work. Mrs. Tapley, referred to as Jean, worked in a general store as a clerk, took care of the inventory, and stocked the shelves. "Does the work of three. Shawn O'Brien, the owner—he works hard too. He's told Jean that if she took time off, she'd lose her job. Jean is well-liked in our small community."

"Can I call Mrs. Tapley at work?" I asked.

"No, she's not allowed to use the phone. You just tell me, and I'll see to it she gets the information. Ours is a poor county, and we only have that one store for groceries. Now, Doctor, don't you be hard on Shawn O'Brien. His earnings from that store ain't much. He's not really a bad man: drinks a bit too much, I'm told—he's a Catholic—but we need that store."

Mrs. Jenkins had sized me up, a big-city doctor; she didn't want me to think poorly of her community, concluding with a nice portrait of Penny's doctor.

"That Doctor Bodey! He gives away more free care than you can imagine. We're both members of the Baptist church," she said proudly.

During the history, Penny sat like a pyramid of flesh, looking at me as if to say, "Don't you dare come near me." I showed her the end of my stethoscope, but she shoved it away with a frown. She didn't retreat to Mrs. Jenkins's arms; she was going to tough this out by herself. I'd have Penny taken to the treatment room, where we'd do a physical exam and then the bone marrow. I sat back in my chair, retreating from her private space.

Penny, a two-year-old, had won round one.

• • •

Dee asked if I would mind working with just one nurse, Morgan. "Of course not," I said. "We'll give it a go. I'm easy, but I think Penny's a two-nurse patient."

Morgan went to get Penny. Ten minutes later Morgan and Brigid entered the treatment room carrying a struggling two-year-old. Morgan had attempted to carry Penny in by herself. Morgan's nurse's cap had been pulled off to one side, and most of her hair hung in her face. Brigid was holding each upper arm, and Morgan was trying to manage the legs. Mrs. Jenkins had helped open the doors but then retreated to Penny's room.

"Well, Doctor H.," Morgan said, "you were right."

"Yes. But once we correct that anemia, she'll be a three-nurse patient."

To be as gentle as possible, it took all three of us to remove her dress. There was a hematoma where blood had been drawn before she was transferred and a protruding abdomen due to her enlarged spleen and liver. The upper half of her body was free of any other lesions, and her fingernails were clean and trimmed.

When we removed Penny's diaper, there was a god-awful smell. Brigid said, "Oh, she needs to be cleaned up. If you'll hold her, Morgan, I'll get a Pampers."

I held Penny's shoulders while Morgan wiped and then washed Penny's bottom. "What's a Pampers?" I asked.

Morgan explained that it was the name of a disposable diaper that had been on the market for a few years. "I gather you're not married and don't have any children, Doctor H."

"No, I'm just an ill-informed internist."

With Penny wearing a fresh Pampers, the three of us completed the evaluation. Penny didn't cry, but she repeatedly yelled no.

The last thing one does when examining an infant is the oral exam. Even a cooperative patient like Michelle Karr cried when a tongue depressor was inserted into her mouth. Penny refused to open her mouth for the exam, and I decided the size of her tonsils could remain a mystery.

The marrow was done with a shriek. I decided to defer the IV until after I had looked at the results.

After thanking both nurses for their help, I suggested that Morgan ask Mrs. Jenkins to come to the treatment room. On seeing her caretaker, Penny put up her arms and was quietly carried out of the soundproof room.

"What a fighter," Brigid said. "Doctor Humphrey, you seemed to be amused by that wrestling match."

"If Michelle Karr is a snuggle bunny, then Penny Tapley's a growling grizzly-bear cub. They're the yin and yang of infancy. I like Penny; she's easy to respect."

"Which one would you rather adopt and take home?" Brigid said with a grin. "Penny or Michelle?"

"Todd Yardley."

Brigid frowned.

"He's housebroken."

• • •

After looking at Penny's marrow and confirming she had ALL, I ran into Morgan in the hall. Her hair and nurse's cap were back in place. "Well, we've found something Penny likes about 2 East. She likes to eat. She doesn't smile; she just eats. She's too young to use food as a bribe. We'll just feed her because she's a neat little girl, even if she's not housebroken."

After entering Penny's room, I sat down and explained leukemia to Mrs. Jenkins, who took notes, asked a few questions, and said she'd be sure Jean got the information that evening.

Finally, I commented on the enlarged abdomen and the big spleen and liver and mentioned that Penny was very clean and someone had bathed her this morning.

"That someone was Jean, Doctor," Mrs. Jenkins said in a short voice. She sat up and continued, "There're kids in town; you can smell 'em before you see 'em. Not Jean's kids. Their clothes may be too big or too small, and the colors may not match, but those three Tapley kids are always clean. Nice kids too. That ten-year-old sister isn't going to run away from home when she's fifteen and get pregnant. Jean does right by those kids."

Out in the hall, I thought, you're full of shit, Humphrey. My middle-class background and my presumptuous feelings about lower classes had just slapped me in the face. I thought, you don't have to have an over-protective mother like Mrs. Paul or two upper-class professional parents like the Thurmans to provide for your kid.

In the Tapley family budget, a bar of soap was probably a significant item.

• • •

At half past one in the afternoon, Morgan and Brigid brought a strug-gling, screaming Penny into the treatment room. Starting an IV is never simple, but for Penny, extra care would be required. After finding a vein, we would tape that arm or leg to an IV board and see if we had truly immobilized the limb. Then I'd clean the skin and attempt to estab-lish IV access. The nurses discussed how they were going to hold Penny. Morgan had good control over the upper half of Penny, and Brigid was doing her best with Penny's legs when, all of a sudden, Morgan let go and said over Penny's shrieking, "She bit me!"

"Brigid, please control Penny. Human bites are nothing to fool around with."

The skin on Morgan's forearm bore the imprint of central incisors, but the skin had not been broken. After I swabbed the site with iodine and then alcohol, I said, "We can't have this happen again. Morgan, please tell Dee we need another pair of hands."

Dee came in herself and organized the holding crew, all out of reach of those teeth.

After finding a vein, I released the tourniquet and taped the entire left arm to a board. Satisfied that Penny's arm was immobilized, I reapplied the tourniquet, and the vein came back into view.

Four adults leaned over a two-year-old, each of us intent on our task. After a blood return on the first stick, I inserted IV tubing into the hub of the needle and taped the tubing to Penny's forearm. I stood up and exhaled.

The nurses loosened their grip on Penny. In a millisecond, Penny's right hand was free from Morgan's grip, and she reached over, grabbed the tubing, and yanked out the IV.

Morgan put her hands up to her face and cried, "Oh no."

Calmly but quickly, Dee took the IV tubing out of Penny's hand, reached over to the IV tray, grabbed a sterile gauze four-by-four, and applied it to the bleeding IV site.

Penny stopped screaming, set her jaw, and looked at each of us with a frown. Morgan was crying and trying to tell me she was sorry. Waving both of my hands to indicate that it was no one's fault, I started to say that Penny had another arm and two legs, but the absurdity of it all resulted in my laughing. Four adults had taken on a two-year-old and lost.

A few minutes passed before I stopped laughing and Morgan stopped crying. Brigid got another IV tray, and Dee kept pressure on the IV site.

"OK, team, let's regroup," I said. After ten minutes, we had another IV going in the other arm.

Penny now had both arms taped to IV boards wrapped in gauze. At the end of each board, down by the hands, were long strips of gauze that could be used to tie the restraints to the crib railings. Thus Penny was forced to lie on her back and prevented from either moving her hands or flipping over and getting tangled in the tubing. Finally, Brigid and Dee carried an exhausted Penny to her room.

"I'm sorry, Doctor Humphrey. I'm surprised you're not angry," Morgan said.

"All three of you should receive the Navy Cross for Valor, and you should also get a Purple Heart for being bitten in the line of duty."

At that absurd analogy, Morgan smiled and blew her nose on a sterile four-by-four from the IV tray.

"Morgan, please sit down. Stay in the treatment room for a few minutes, and I'll be right back." Three minutes later, I returned. "I thought you might like a cup of coffee, Morgan."

• • •

My rounds Thursday morning went off without a hitch. First, Penny's IV was still working. She was not febrile, her hemoglobin had been partially corrected, and the uric-acid level was within normal limits. Furthermore, she had eaten a good breakfast and hadn't bitten anyone. Not a bad start.

Having learned something yesterday and not wanting to make another social blunder, I took a quick inventory of any biases I might be harboring about low-income families. I found one: don't assume that Mrs. Tapley could not fully understand the complexities of leukemia.

When I walked down to Penny's room, I found a big sign on the door.

Be Careful
Penny Bites

I smiled and waited a minute for the humor of the sign to wear off. A fleeting image ran through my mind: this not being a hospital room but a cage at the zoo. I knocked on the door, went over to Penny, said a few words, and then sat down in front of Mrs. Jenkins.

"Jean understands the diagnosis." Mrs. Jenkins looked at some notes. She had only two questions: "Is Penny going to get better?" "Is Penny going to die?"

Wow! Penny's mom had the courage to ask that second question. The first was relatively easy to answer: yes. The concept of a remission was explained to Mrs. Jenkins. The answer to the second question: "We don't know."

Mrs. Jenkins seemed to understand it was too early to know how effective POMP was going to be.

"To be honest, we already know it isn't going to cure everyone, but we hoped it might cure a few."

"Well, Doctor, that's what we'll hope and pray for."

Walking back to the nurses' station, I thought, for Penny I'd be willing to get down on my own knees if I believed there was the remotest chance that it would do any good.

• • •

"Is something wrong?" Mrs. Jenkins asked.

"Oh no," I said. "I often just stop by to see how things are going. It's a habit. In some rooms, there are puzzles to put together, and in other rooms there's time to talk of dogs."

Mrs. Jenkins didn't have any questions. I was almost out the door when I turned and asked, "Do you think Doctor Bodey would mind if I called him?"

"You go right ahead. He'll want to know about Penny. We don't know how he does it. That man has time for everyone."

Calling Doctor Bodey's office and introducing myself to his nurse, I said I didn't want to interrupt and asked when he'd be free to take a phone call about Penny Tapley. She told me he wanted to talk to me now.

Doctor Bodey listened to a few comments on the diagnosis and the treatment plan. When I tried to compliment him on making the diagnosis, his jovial response was, "I miss a lot of things too, but folks around here seem to forgive me." What he really wanted to know was

131

how Penny was. When I told him she was OK, a feisty little girl, he said, "That's our Penny."

When I said that I was sorry that NIH didn't have a mechanism to pay for his office visits, he laughed. "A lot of folks around here don't have money to pay my bills, but many of my patients stop by with baskets of fresh vegetables or fruits, smoked hams, chickens, canned fruits, and all sorts of things. I've been getting fat for years on these types of payment." He asked me to spell my name and gave me his home phone number.

That night at the fence, I told Domino that my phone call to Doctor Bodey had transported me back to a childhood fantasy. One of my childhood heroes was my pediatrician, Doctor Sidney Sinclair Snyder. His office was on the second floor over a pharmacy on South Ninety-Fifth Street and full of jars containing cotton balls, gauze, fluids, and pills. He made house calls, like when I had chicken pox, and opened up his office nights and weekends, like the time I had a small laceration of my skull, the result of trying to give my sister a piggyback ride.

As a five-year-old, I decided to be a general practitioner in a small community, a pillar of society, delivering babies and watching them grow up. It never occurred to me that anyone in my care would die. Here I was, on the bottom rung of the most important medical research institute in the world, a thirty-year-old with an MD and PhD who had fantasies of doing research in molecular biology. Now I was responsible for very sick patients who would never grow up.

"You know, Domino, I respect Doctor Bodey, but I don't envy him. He has a different kind of hard work to accomplish each day. He's available all week and every weekend for the birth of an infant to the care of the elderly: a womb-to-tomb practice. I don't know how he does it."

Domino nuzzled me for his carrot.

• • •

"Ben, are you dating anyone, have a girl back home, anything like that?" Jerry asked.

"Well," I said, "there were a few dates with an attractive divorcée in July and August, but that didn't last. I'm corresponding with a graduate student in Mainz, but nothing's certain, and I still think about a great girl from my last year in grad school."

"Good," he said. "I also don't date divorcees; what that German babe doesn't know won't hurt her, and we all make mistakes. So you're free. You need to do something other than ride that damn horse."

Jerry was dating someone who had a girlfriend named Sheila. He had met her and went on and on about her figure. She was "built," "r-e-a-l-l-y built," and he thought she would be "easy." He had taken the liberty to tell her about me and said I might call. "I hope you don't mind."

"Of course not. I'll call her this evening."

On Thursday, I told Jerry, "We have a date on Saturday night."

• • •

I arrived at six o'clock at Sheila's apartment and was met at the door by a strawberry blonde.

Sheila had a pleasant manner and smile and wore a red-velvet mini-dress and matching boots. Her ample body was characterized by curves, curves everywhere with no suggestion of her being overweight.

We started out in one of Jerry's favorite bars. The place was full of miniskirts, boots, and long eyelashes. Guys wore Beatles-type suits or black turtleneck sweaters, and I felt absolutely naked without a peace button.

Dinner passed quietly, with many pleasant exchanges. Shelia wanted to know about living in Germany.

"Let me tell you about a memorable evening. I was at a party of about twenty students. Someone turned off the music, and a student announced that President Kennedy had been assassinated. There was dead silence. Everybody got up and went home."

Sheila told me she'd been in a bar when she learned of Kennedy's death. Then in a reflective mood, she said, "The German students showed that much respect for our president." Then she added, "I guess I shouldn't be surprised. He gave that famous speech in Berlin: 'Ich bin ein Berliner.'"

When I asked if she wanted to go for a walk after dinner, Shelia said no and that she wasn't feeling well. "Bad timing. I really enjoyed the evening, Ben. Makes me think I ought to try a European holiday."

It was easy for me to echo her comment about the evening.

I slowly drove back to Kirkhill. To my surprise, Thomas Kuhn's *The Structure of Scientific Revolutions* came to mind. He got it right: "People from different paradigms can't converse." But, I thought, they could spend a pleasant evening together talking about the worlds they lived in.

Third Week

There were no problems on 2 East, so Rick talked about a few domestic issues on Monday morning. Jerry elected to pass and looked at me. "Well?"

Jerry explained to Rick that he had fixed me up.

"Shelia was attractive, pleasant company and was full-figured as you promised. The restaurant was excellent, and we talked about a number of things," I said, summarizing our evening together.

"Ah," Jerry said, "the bars of Georgetown are full of good-looking chicks, but I picked this one out for you. When are you going to see her again?"

Rick got up and went to see a patient, apparently not interested in listening to two bachelors in delayed adolescence discuss women.

"Despite an interesting evening, no future plans."

"Why not?"

"Well, it's a question of two different people from two different worlds. Sheila's not going to go out and buy English riding attire, nor should she. I'm not going to get a Beatles suit. Sheila likes to party, and I need to talk to a horse."

And then Jerry blew me away. "You're not going to believe this, but when we had lunch with Jody and Rick to celebrate their starting a family, I was a little jealous: Rick had found someone, and he was getting on with his life."

"No, Jerry," I said, "I believe you." I too felt emptiness in my personal life. But now was not the time to ponder this, with patients to take care of.

• • •

This Monday morning, there were two third-week names on the Board as expected: Robert "Gosh" Thurman and Billy "Bear" Sullivan.

This was Robert's second admission. I hoped that his parents could continue to alternate staying with him. I enjoyed seeing a father on the floor, and I wanted to hear about the puppy that had joined the family.

Billy and Mrs. Sullivan were seasoned veterans of 2 East. Hopefully Billy's much-beloved teddy bear would not be encrusted with blood from a nosebleed.

If they were both in remission, I thought, it should be a delightful week.

• • •

"You'd better see Robert first, Doctor Humphrey," Brigid said. "I've been in his room a couple of times, and each time he asked if you were on the floor. He's got a picture he wants to show you."

I thanked her and walked down to Robert's room. Before I could say good morning, he hopped off the bed and said, "Here."

Pretending not to look at it immediately, I thanked him. "I bet it's a picture of your soccer team."

"Nooo. It's my new puppy."

What a way to start the day. Robert was onto my attempt to tease him. I was then treated to a refreshing stream of information. Of greatest importance was that the puppy didn't have a name. Robert was going to live with his pet for a few weeks, "to see what name fit."

Dad and Mom were both present. They were both anxious. Did their son respond to POMP? Was he in remission? A very small percent of patients would not go into remission. They knew it, and so did I.

At 10:05 a.m., I returned from the path lab. "Robert's in remission."

Robert's dad smiled, and his mother said through a flood of tears, "I knew he'd make it."

Later in the day, Mr. Thurman was taking his turn while his wife was at work. I asked if he'd mind if I took Robert up to the path lab to look at some marrow cells. He agreed, and when I said, "Robert, we're going to a laboratory to look down a microscope at your marrow," I got my first gosh of the afternoon. Robert skipped and danced all the way up to the path lab. As we looked down the microscope together, he bombarded me with a series of goshes. Robert now had images to remember for the new terms he was learning.

• • •

Monday mornings were never routine, but my exchanges with some of my little patients fell into a pattern. When I walked into his room, Billy extended Bear to me with both hands. I sat down on the edge of Billy's bed, and I said hello to Mrs. Sullivan. We boys played with Bear, and I did my pretend physical exam. I looked at a couple of Billy's books, opening one about an Indian boy and his canoe.

Showing Billy the picture, I asked, "What is this?"

"Canoe," said Billy, and I raised my eyebrows.

Mrs. Sullivan explained that his uncle lived on a small lake. "If there's no wind, Billy is wrapped up in a life preserver, firmly held in the front of the canoe by his dad while his uncle paddles. He loves that canoe," she said, "so I bought him that book."

At half past ten, I returned from the treatment room carrying a sobbing Billy. He normally did not sit on his mother's lap, but after a bone-marrow aspiration he welcomed her comforting arms.

At 11:10, I was back in Billy's room with the good news of another remission.

"I also like to canoe, but where I go, there are real live bears, and they can steal your food while you're sleeping in your tent."

"Is that the canoe country in northern Minnesota?" Mrs. Sullivan asked.

"Yes, I often escaped from my graduate studies to go camping and canoeing."

Looking at Mrs. Sullivan, I thought, it's too bad we can't send mothers up into bear country to escape. Bears are scary but not as frightening as POMP.

● ● ●

On Tuesday-morning rounds, I told Jay that Billy was in remission and receiving POMP, and Robert Thurman was also on schedule.

As Jerry explained the status of a patient who had just relapsed, the sea got a little rough. "The parents are now considering whether to go ahead with a trial of daunomycin. They're home and going to meet with their priest. I did my best and even mentioned Jimmy Paul."

To his credit, Jay didn't say, "What the hell does a priest know about leukemia?" Instead he suggested that, in the future, the priest or minister might be encouraged to visit the Clinical Center.

Jerry defended his decision to let the family go home to decide about daunomycin. Then, in a soft, slow voice he said, "It is their child, after all."

God, I loved Jerry for saying that. In his corner, Rick nodded.

Jay leaned back in his chair. "That's right."

As the year went on, I continued to wonder, how many sides of his personality did Jay keep in reserve? How many were necessary to work on 2 East, to survive being on 2 East, and to be willing to return to 2 East, year after year? A bigger question for me was, was I acquiring a new way of being? New value judgments?

• • •

Both Jerry and I wanted to listen to Rick explain how in Minnesota he went about presenting a phase II trial to a mother at the time of relapse. Since July 1, two patients had relapsed, and both mothers did not accept a trial of daunomycin.

"I've got a mom in front of me whose kid has just been through the hell of POMP. What do I say to her?" Jerry asked.

"Being on POMP is different from the phase III trials that we used in Minnesota. Two drugs for induction and two drugs for maintenance. There was less toxicity. Furthermore, we didn't make a big deal out of phase II. It was more like, the leukemia is back, and this is the next drug to try to get rid of it."

"So, we don't know why a mother *would* choose to try daunomycin. I've got an idea," I said. "John Billingsworth, the clinical associate from last year, got Jimmy Paul into the phase II protocol. I'll talk to him and get back to you guys."

I made arrangements to meet John in his research lab. We exchanged bits of information about our backgrounds, his current research, and my plans for next year. When I asked how he had convinced Mrs. Paul to participate in the daunomycin phase II trial, he smiled.

"You don't convince Mrs. Paul of anything," he said. "She knew about the protocol and wanted Jimmy to receive the drug."

"Do you know why?

"No."

Before I left, John asked how a few specific patients were doing. I filled him in and said I would extend his regards to the mothers.

After passing this information on to Jerry and Rick, they both wanted me to call Mrs. Paul. I was the only one who had a speaking acquaintance with a mother who had accepted a phase II agent.

I thought, be careful. The mothers of 2 East know things that aren't in the toxicity section of the POMP protocol.

It wasn't my habit to interview a patient or a mother, and I wanted to think ahead about my conversation with Mrs. Paul. I wouldn't be able to observe facial expressions or body language to judge if Mrs. Paul was uncomfortable talking to me about her time at NIH. I had never interviewed a patient or a mother over the phone, and I wanted to think ahead about my conversation with Mrs. Paul. I thought, when you call, proceed in a friendly but orderly manner. So as not to digress or forget something, I made a list:

1. *Ask if it's OK to talk.*
2. *Comments on liking Jimmy. That would be easy for me.*
3. *Mention that you recently talked to John Billingsworth.*
4. *State the reason for the phone call. Play it straight. Ask her why she chose to have Jimmy receive the drug.*
5. *Finally thank her and ask if she has any questions.*

Mrs. Paul answered the phone. Although she was still adjusting to Jimmy's death, she said she didn't mind my calling.

The conversation proceeded without difficulty. The answer to why she agreed to the daunomycin was, "I didn't want any what-ifs haunting me. We tried it, and it didn't work, but Jimmy probably lived a little longer, four months longer." She felt the toxicity was unpleasant but reminded me, "Jimmy was a tough little boy."

My response came easily: "He was indeed."

"You know, Doctor, when your child is four years old, four months is a lot of time."

• • •

Dee knocked on the office door, came in, and handed Jerry a letter. "It's from Betty's mother, Helen Miller. I'm sure she'd like you to see it."

Jerry took a sheet of paper out of the envelope and read it slowly, refolded it, and then came over to my desk. "I think you ought to see this, Ben. You also spent time with Betty."

Dear Dee,

I want to thank you and all the nurses for the loving care you gave Betty and the support you gave to me during Betty's illness.

During this past month, we have been blessed with kind words from members of our church. They mean well, but they were not at the bedside like you and the rest of the nurses.

I have decided not to change anything in Betty's bedroom. I go in there every night. It's a place to remember my little girl and cry. God blessed me with a loving child for two years.

Please tell Doctor Sandler I appreciate all they did for Betty. Also thank the other two doctors.

You, Barbara, and everyone are in my prayers.

God bless you,
Helen Miller

"I think Rick..." I swallowed. "I think Rick should also see this."

Rick read the letter later. "The issue of the bedroom is very difficult for many mothers," he said. "After the death, we made a specific appointment with the moms and said they would be welcome to return, but they didn't have to. We learned a lot from those mothers."

Jerry stopped writing in a chart, and I put a medical journal down.

"I guess about a third came back," Rick said. "From some moms, just passing by the bedroom was difficult. They approached the problem in several ways. Some set a specific date to clean out the room. Some moms needed a sister or close friend to help. Clothes were mostly given to Goodwill; toys and books were often donated to our waiting room."

"Dee told me about the toys in our playroom," Jerry said.

"I want to tell you about a specific adolescent," Rick said. "He was especially proud of his room, and before he died, he asked that his mother not change anything for one year. Then he wanted it cleaned out. He instructed her on a few of his possessions that he wanted to go to specific friends. At the end of that year, when she cleaned out his room, she found a letter addressed to her saying he loved her, he was OK, and that he wanted her to be OK."

● ● ●

"There's a letter for you," Frank said when I got home.

"While there's still some light in the evening sky, I think I'll lunge Whirley-Wee."

"It's from Germany," Frank added.

"Thanks. Probably from a friend or Professor Siebert, the head of the lab in Mainz."

"It's from *Kristina*."

"Oh. In that case, I'll open it," I said.

Frank and I both dated a number of girls while we roomed together in Chicago, but we rarely commented on these relationships. If Frank wanted to know about Kristina, I was more than willing to tell him.

"Would you like to see a picture of Kristina?"

"Yes," Frank said emphatically.

Rummaging through a stack of photos, I found two photographs of Kristina. The first was from a student Bavarian ski vacation in December when I met her. The second was from the Neiderwald, the forest above Rüdesheim, where we often hiked on weekends. On these hikes, Kristina wore a peasant costume, a dirndl-style dress with a long black skirt. A hand-embroidered apron added color to the costume, and the darker color of the dress accentuated her blond hair.

"Wow," Frank said. "What a striking Fräulein. Tell me about her."

"She's a graduate student in linguistics, and her home was in Freiburg. I visited her parents, and it was very clear that her mother didn't like me. She had a son living in England, she said, and that was enough. Because Kristina had lived in England, her English is extremely good. When my parents visited me in Mainz, they met Kristina."

"Am I going to meet this Fräulein?"

"I don't know. We had talked about her coming to America next year."

I didn't tell Frank that I had a few reservations about Kristina. She was almost *too* good-looking. She might be more like a trophy or a souvenir. Earlier, I had thought of a ski vacation in Europe this winter but had already begun to realize that going to Europe wasn't very likely because of 2 East. While Rick and Jerry would gladly cover for me, this wasn't a year for escaping.

Fourth Week

At a quarter to eight in the morning, I was looking at the Board. There were three names listed for me, my happy trio. The baby, Michelle Karr, was my snuggle bunny. Preadolescent girl Tammy Long was my pied beauty with her overabundance of makeup and perfume. Finally, Todd Yardley, who was full of surprises; in July it was stories about his dog, Ralph, and in August it was a collection of canine riddles. What would Todd have for me today?

Michelle sat on my lap for a few minutes, and Tammy was as pretty as ever and still shy when I complimented her on her makeup, but it was Todd who surprised me with an exuberant greeting.

"Supercalifragilisticexpialidocious," Todd yelled as I walked into his room.

I raised my eyebrows. Todd repeated his greeting. I shrugged.

Brigid was also in the room, taking Todd's pulse.

"Can you translate that into English?" I asked Brigid.

"No, nor can I repeat whatever it is," she said with a smile.

Mrs. Yardley suggested that Todd repeat the word and break it down into parts. "Then, Brigid and Doctor Humphrey can learn it."

So Brigid and I, presumably two individuals of above-average intelligence, took instructions from a five-year-old on how to say *supercalifragilisticexpialidocious.*

It took a number of trials before we got it down to Todd's satisfaction. Brigid could pronounce it after the third practice session, but it took me at least five attempts to get it almost perfect.

"It's from *Mary Poppins*, a film by Walt Disney," Mrs. Yardley explained. "Very enjoyable for both kids and adults—stars Julie Andrews."

"Go see it!" Todd commanded.

"If you two are going to take care of kids, you'd better see this film. It's been out for a few weeks, but don't go to a matinee or even the early show."

I accompanied Brigid as she left the room and asked if she would like to see the movie with me Saturday night. She smiled and said yes.

As I watched her walk back to the nurses' station, I thought, wow. That was sudden and spontaneous on your part, Humphrey. Where was the usual analysis about asking a girl for a date? Was the spontaneity of the way my little patient acted altering me? Oh well, I had a new word and a date with a pleasant, attractive young woman. A five-year-old had said, "Go see it."

• • •

A tail thumping against the foot of my bed woke me from a sound sleep. A wet nose greeted me; Shonto wanted to go out, and she didn't care who responded. As Frank was still asleep, I got up, opened the front door, and went to the kitchen.

On this September morn, the temperature was mild, the sun not yet overhead. Too early to play the water-tank game but not too early for sweet feed and hay, Domino trotted up to the fence; the Thoroughbreds followed suit. All was well in my rural world, bucolic even, as all of my trio had been discharged on Friday.

Sitting on the bench by the barn, I gazed at the Maryland countryside; some of the oaks were yellow, and the sumac was red, an occasional milkweed seed floating by. My empty head allowed me to take all of this in. Being empty is very different from being drained, and this morning, I was aware of the difference. Savor the moment, I thought.

We put up the hay that had been delivered, its musty odor suffusing the air. Then Frank and I spent most of the morning riding. We now had reasonably well-trained three-gaited saddle horses. To get our Thoroughbreds used to different riders, we often swapped mounts, just in case either of us wanted to take a guest riding. Frank's Galla-B was easier to handle, but Whirley-Wee had smoother gaits. The horses had been worked up to a sweat, another special and favorite aroma.

Lunch was a thick slice of virginia ham on rye bread, lettuce, tomato, mayonnaise, and a dill pickle. It was just warm enough for a cold beer. Thereafter, I indulged in a nap under the tree by the barn.

After cleaning up, I left Kirkhill in the early evening for my date with Brigid to see *Mary Poppins*. We had agreed to go to the late show at eight o'clock and avoid the long lines.

Arriving at her apartment on Wisconsin Avenue at seven, I wasn't prepared for the Brigid that opened the door. She was wearing a black cotton dress and dark stockings. Brigid was tall, probably five seven or eight, and wore pumps with a medium heel. Her long brown hair was pulled back in a french roll. She was wearing a light-red lipstick and maybe a bit of rouge. "That's a very becoming outfit," I said. Before this evening, I had only seen Brigid in a nurse's uniform. She knew I was a bit surprised.

"Thank you," she said. "It's also nice to see you in a blazer and not a white coat."

I had the top up on the Healey so as not to disturb her hair. As I helped her into the car, I noticed a faint aroma of a musk-like perfume. After months of enjoying the odor of a horse, now there was the sweet smell of a woman.

We waited in line for twenty minutes before seating started. There were a few young couples in line but mostly parents with school-age children. Brigid laughed when I told her that we should have asked Mrs. Yardley to borrow Todd so we wouldn't seem out of place. We passed the time exchanging information on backgrounds and various hobbies. I asked Brigid not to address me as Doctor. She agreed but rarely called me Ben.

After the film, we went for coffee.

"What song did you like the best?" I asked.

"That's easy for me," Brigid said. "'A Spoonful of Sugar.' Too bad life isn't that simple. And you?"

"Well, 'Supercalifragilisticexpialidocious' was fun, and we should remember that's what got us to see the film, but I liked 'Feed the Birds' the most."

"Ah yes," Brigid said. "And do you feed birds? Do you have a bird feeder where you live?"

"No. I feed horses," I said and also told her about Squirrel.

After I escorted her to her apartment, we agreed it had been a fun evening and decided to do something together again.

That night at the fence, I gave everybody two carrots. It had been a pleasant day, a relaxing day. I wondered if this was how normal people spent their weekends.

OCTOBER

First Week

Monday morning. Some people read the headlines of the *Washington Post*; some listened to the news on their car radio as they drove to work; I looked at the Board in the nurses' station on 2 East. Two names: Sarah Thompkins, my honest six-year-old, and John Graham, my withdrawn eleven-year-old. I sighed. I thought about the school program that his mother had told me about last month. A school psychologist was going to work with him and meet regularly with his parents. I hoped there would be good news.

• • •

Sarah was her normal cooperative self and as usual made it clear she wasn't happy to see me. Mrs. Thompkins was a little less laconic and commented she was eager to see Julia Graham.

By a quarter to ten, I was able to tell Sarah she was in remission. "You tell your doctor thank you," Mrs. Thompkins commanded, and Sarah complied.

I told her she was welcome and that I was pleased too. No response from Sarah, and I thought, I love this little girl.

• • •

"I'm sorry we're late, Doctor Humphrey," Mrs. Graham said, "but I just couldn't get organized this morning."

"It's only ten fifteen. No problem."

I suggested we get the bad stuff over with before lunch and told Mrs. Graham, "We can talk about John's school program during rest period."

"That'll be fine."

Her expressionless affect told me the work with the school psychologist hadn't been a roaring success. Mrs. Graham seemed haggard, and I wondered if she had lost weight.

At a quarter to noon, I could tell John, in his mother's presence, that there were no bad cells in his marrow—only good ones.

Lunch on my bench under the tree at 12:40 p.m. gave me an opportunity to talk to my buddy Squirrel. "The mechanics of treatment seem to be working, but somehow something's very wrong."

Squirrel sat on his haunches and munched a peanut.

During the rest hour, Mrs. Graham summarized John's response to the school program: there was no major improvement. The school psychologist, Doctor White, had not given up hope on John recovering from the trauma he had experienced. Dr. White felt that it was important to keep on with the weekly parental meeting.

"There's a new problem at home," Mrs. Graham said. "John's dad is trying to help him fall asleep; he's staying in John's bedroom most of the night. John's father thinks John Junior is having nightmares." Finally she said, "Nothing seems to be working."

I leaned forward and opened my hands. "How is your husband holding up? How are you doing?"

"We support each other. It's a good marriage; I'm sleeping a little better, but I don't have much of an appetite."

"Other than you, does your husband have someone to talk to?"

"His father. Oh, let me tell you about John's grandfather, my father-in-law. He's a wonderful man; we always enjoy his visits. Before John was sick, the three Graham men would do things together. John really liked and talked about it for months after each visit."

"That reminds me of my childhood," I said. "Please go on."

"Well, Granddad spent three days with us two weeks ago. During his visit, he and John spent time together." Mrs. Graham went into a few details. "My father-in-law rarely speaks to anyone about his experiences in World War I, especially the time he spent in the trenches, yet at the end of his visit, he said John reminded him of one of his comrades who suffered shell shock."

It was 1964; Grandfather Graham was way ahead of his time. Years later, shell shock would be called posttraumatic stress disorder or PTSD. Finally in 1987, the Diagnostic and Statistical Manual of Mental Disorders published by the American Psychiatric Association, the infamous DSM, would list children as being at risk for PSTD.

• • •

Over coffee, Rick and I talked about John. After describing the sequence of events, I sighed. "I feel helpless."

Rick shrugged. "I don't know, Ben. Sometimes, I don't think anything I learned, experienced, or was taught in Minnesota is helping me here on 2 East. Did you talk to Myron about John?"

"Yeah. That was the one bright spot last month. Myron said he'd have a social worker from the disclosure program spend time with John. Nothing was learned, but despite this, Mrs. Graham appreciated the effort. She told me, 'You're trying, the school's trying, everybody is trying, and maybe something will come of all this effort.'"

• • •

Thursday morning, a quarter past ten. Jerry came into the office and sat down with a plunk. "Goddamn! Another case of fever and a low white count."

Closing the journal I was reading, I said, "I'm going to see Myron."

Myron invited me into his office. "I need a break. What's up, Ben?"

"Well, there is some hostility about the toxicity of POMP among the clinical associates on 2 East," I said. "The scuttlebutt is that an LD10 was written into the POMP protocol. Now, I never heard of the LD or lethal-dose concept during my residency or during med school."

"The concept is simple enough," Myron said. "You keep escalating the dose of a drug in mice until a specific dose kills ten out of a hundred animals. When starting a new drug in humans, the initial dose is significantly below the LD10 for mice, or dogs."

"Yeah, I know; I've had to learn about that here at NIH. But when it comes to combining drugs, how do you do that? Does Jay Freireich write an LD10 into the protocol?"

Sighing deeply, Myron reminded me that I lacked the historical perspective of the chemotherapy that preceded POMP. "Jay and Tom were evaluating two drug combinations in the late 1950s and four drug combinations *for the last four years*. But they took a lot of heat from people like Max Wintrobe when they started."

"The author of *Clinical Hematology*? The big standard text."

"Yeah. A self-proclaimed expert on leukemia. Max said something like the drugs cause more harm than good and shouldn't be used. At any rate, the drugs do work; we got kids living for over a year and a few off therapy. First there was VAMP, started in 1962; then BIKE in 1963; and now POMP, which started in January 1964. So you see, a lot of experience went into designing POMP."

"OK, OK. But patients are still experiencing low white-blood-cell counts and occasionally develop sepsis."

Careful with his choice of words, Myron said, "Jay's tough; he's willing to write a protocol that will produce severe neutropenia. He believes you can treat sepsis with antibiotics but you can't treat a relapse. But Jay didn't sit down and plan to write a drug schedule that would be so toxic it would kill ten percent of the patients. There's a big difference between the two." Myron paused and let the message sink in. "We look at clinical responses of patients on POMP weekly. And every week, we ask, is it too much therapy?"

"What else do you guys do for entertainment?" I quipped.

"You son of a bitch," Myron retorted. "Go play with some mice, and let us try to do something of potential value."

"Oh, you never go into the laboratory? To be honest, your comments on toxicity have been helpful. May I share them with Rick and Jerry?"

"Of course! Why not?"

"You're one of the big dogs around here, and I'm just a fire hydrant. When I get pissed on by Jay, that's my problem, and I don't come whining to you."

"I appreciate that," Myron said. "You're not a fire hydrant, but you are a little wet behind the ears."

I chuckled and then leaned back in the chair and frowned.

"There's something else bothering you, isn't there?"

"Every now and then, especially before going to bed, I wonder if there is any difference between a patient dying from leukemia and a patient dying from toxicity. Sometimes, there's no answer. Mostly, the answer is that it's more acceptable for the patient to die of the disease. But maybe it's just a head game. Pondering the cause of a death rather than feeling the tragedy."

"Welcome to the club. We write words on a page, sweat over doses, and ask for biostatistical help. We look at data, and you and the other associates look at patients."

I shrugged. "That's our job."

Myron put his hands behind his head and leaned back. "I'll share with you something that occasionally comes to me. Would I be willing to write an LD20 protocol if I knew it would cure ten percent of the children entered in the study? You kill twenty and cure ten, and the other seventy die of leukemia. When you're passing out carrots tonight, you might wrestle with that."

I thanked Myron for his time and walked back to 2 East. It was an interesting question—one that should be asked in the dark.

• • •

For the horses, it was a two-carrot night as I pondered Myron's provocative question. Nothing consistent flashed through my mind. Just more concerns, questions, and thoughts. More head stuff. As an undergraduate at the University of Wisconsin, I'd taken a course in logic. It was all about "if all of *A* is not *B*" and so on. That translated to, the only way you could be assured that no one died of toxicity was to let everyone die of leukemia. The only way to make sure no one died of leukemia was to use lethal chemotherapy. But leukemia and death occurred in pediatric patients. Reducing all this to *A* and *B* seemed like a bunch of bullshit.

The Thoroughbreds returned to grazing in the dim light of late evening. Domino remained at the fence. He knew what he wanted.

I didn't know it then, but within four years I would write my first pediatric chemotherapy protocols for ALL, wrestle with doses and sequence of administration, and then watch patients relapse. I would still be wrestling with these same problems of toxicity and cures for most of my career.

• • •

The next day, over coffee, the three of us discussed recent publications from the medical literature on childhood leukemia. Rick explained that there were three cooperative groups working on leukemia in children: Leukemia Group A, Leukemia Group B, and the Southwest Oncology Group. Each group consisted of approximately twenty universities. They wrote protocols for the group and thus were able to complete a study much faster than a single institution.

Before we got into much of a discussion, Jay came up to our table and asked if he could join us. "Of course," we chorused.

When Jerry asked about the relative lack of toxicity in therapeutic trials in pediatric leukemia, Jay reminded us that at the average university there was only one individual responsible for both pediatric hematology and oncology. "Some so-called oncologists won't use a toxic schedule; many hematologists will refuse to even consider a toxic protocol. These are the compromises of the cooperative groups."

When Rick asked Jay for his assessment of multi-institutional cooperative groups, Jay quickly came to their defense. Having a command of the literature, he gave examples from recent publications. Furthermore, he told us about studies that had been completed and were currently in press. Finally he told us of research currently in progress, citing the studies he thought most interesting. "These studies are the promise of the cooperative groups," Jay said.

When Jay stood up to leave, Jerry said he appreciated Jay's thoughts. Collecting our photocopies of published papers, we threw them into a stack and turned our attention to drinking coffee.

For me, far more valuable than the data Jay had summarized was his method of keeping on top of his research. As a graduate student, I was encouraged to and did read the literature. More important, I was sent to national scientific congresses to hear scientists summarize, in fifteen minutes, research that they had just completed. But I never thought of keeping track of research in my field of interest that was in progress in other laboratories.

My graduate studies didn't include exposure to drug trials. Now my day was steeped in such research. If I ever needed or wanted to design a clinical study, there was a hell of a lot more to it than I had previously realized.

I had just learned something that even an internist educated at one of the more prestigious universities needed to know. And it was from Jay no less.

● ● ●

Friday's sign-out rounds were relaxed. None of our patients were toxic; no one had died.

"Jerry, last week you used two words," Rick said. "I wrote them down: one was *quaker* or something like that, and the other *miseltop*. I don't think that's quite right either."

Jerry laughed. "Are you enjoying learning some Yiddish, Rick?"

"Yeah. Jody often asks if I've learned any new words."

Jerry explained. *Quaker* was *kvetcher*, a complainer. His English was accent-free, but when telling Yiddish jokes, he could break into a New York manner of expression that always embellished the humor. He made Rick repeat *kvetcher* until he got it right, and Jerry went on to explain that *miseltop* was *mazel tov* and meant congratulations, not for an idea but when something had been completed. Again he made Rick practice the pronunciation. They even did hand gestures to go with both words.

Watching these two, I was in stiches. "We'll have to get you a yarmulke, Rick."

Second Week

Monday's Board announced the happy week of listening to Sally Carter, my "charming chatterbox," and the challenge of caring for Penny "the Biter" Tapley. Mrs. Carter was always a pleasure to listen to with her cordial manner and southern accent. Penny would be accompanied by Mrs. Jenkins. I liked her.

Each month, I looked at Sally Carter's height and weight. During the last three months, Sally had grown an inch taller and gained an additional kilo. This wouldn't have seemed noteworthy for a pediatrician; growth is one of the things most three-year-olds do very well. An internist makes note of a decrease in muscle mass and a decrease in height due to some vertebral compression. Aging is something adults don't always do very well.

Breaking Little Bones

Mrs. Carter kept track of Sally's physical and mental development and, if questioned, could tell me how high Sally could count and new colors she'd learned.

The news this morning was good; Sally was still in remission.

• • •

Penny was in her crib with the railings raised. A stout middle-aged woman greeted me with, "Are you the doctor that treats Penny?" After I nodded, she handed me a few sheets of paper and continued. "Virginia Jenkins told me that the nurses took good care of Penny, so I'll not be staying. I'll pick her up on Friday midday."

The notes the volunteer left were helpful and interesting. Doctor Bodey had made a house call the first day Penny was home and gave Penny's mom a thermometer. Doctor Bodey also made a weekly house call.

I was sorry that I wouldn't have Mrs. Jenkins to chat with during the week. She was proud of her work as a volunteer and of her community and made me aware of the fine attributes of Penny's mom, Jean Tapley, and their community's Doctor Bodey.

Throughout the two-nurse physical exam, Penny was gently held, but during the three-nurse marrow aspiration, everybody was intent on his or her task. Three nurses gritted their teeth, and three pairs of hands firmly and aggressively pinned Peggy to the table. Dee even said, "Dammit, Penny: hold still." I didn't know Dee used these terms, but restraining Penny was not for the faint of heart.

I set my jaw and thrust the needle through the skin, periosteum, and bone with a quick stroke. Pulling the needle out, I said, "We're done." A coda of sighs ended this intense performance. The aggressive grasping was changed to a gentle holding of Penny to keep her on the table. In dealing with Penny, no one got angry; it was more like we all lost our humanity for a few minutes.

I called Doctor Bodey and told him Penny was in remission. He thanked me, said he was pleased, and told me to phone anytime.

Call Mrs. Jenkins, I thought. She answered the phone. "Right nice of you to call, Doctor. You jest let me know if I can run any messages to Jean or Doctor Bodey. Last Sunday, our pastor mentioned Penny in his weekly prayer. It's a special prayer, Doctor, for the good keeping of the members of our church."

I was glad I had spoken with Mrs. Jenkins. That prayer was more than just for Penny's "good keeping." It acknowledged that Penny Tapley was a member of the congregation, and everybody would pray not only for her recovery but her safe return to where she belonged.

• • •

During Monday's lunch, the three of us discussed whether we needed to send someone down to another clinic on Tuesday morning to buy a couple of days for the patient to recover from POMP.

Rick and I felt our admissions were just routine-risk patients.

Jerry had a candidate, a six-year-old girl named Mary, to whom he had given four days of IV antibiotics the previous month after she completed POMP. She was again admitted with a low white count and presumably hadn't fully recovered.

We all agreed that Jerry's patient was at the greatest risk and therefore there would be no POMP today and tomorrow. Tuesday morning Mary would be in the ENT clinic because she had pain in an ear.

I had admitted both Penny "the Biter" Tapley and Sally "Doctor Humpfee" Carter. Of my two patients, it was Sally who concerned me. For each of the previous three admissions, her white count on admission had been quite low, yet she had never developed a fever that required blood cultures and IV antibiotics.

Sally's low white count was a number on a slip of paper—a high-risk laboratory finding, but my response was emotional. I was trying to avoid thinking about a relapse of leukemia in my beautiful little chatterbox.

• • •

There was a lot to think about as I drove home to Kirkhill. The three of us had reluctantly decided to protect one of Jerry's patients. "Protect" was a nice way of referring to a protocol violation.

As I walked toward the fence with three carrots, I knew I was still haunted by the violence of obtaining Penny's marrow. Penny was in remission, but I wasn't. It would take a day or two for my feelings of having been that aggressive with a child to abate.

But then I thought, if one assumes things are either growing or declining, then Rick, as a pediatrician, was specializing in growth and development, and I, as an internist, was specializing in decay and decline. I wasn't aware that, subconsciously, I was beginning to wonder if that was really the path I wanted to take.

• • •

Tuesday-morning rounds. My patients and Rick's patients were on schedule. Freireich didn't challenge Jerry about his patient getting an ENT consult for an earache.

When Freireich left the doctors' office, Rick and I smiled, and Jerry let out a long sigh.

Jerry quipped that our "Monday Noon Risk Conference" was "The Jennifer Johnson Memorial Hour." Then there was Jerry's Betty Miller, and in a mordant moment, I called it the "Let's Try to Keep Everybody

Waving Conference." We took the decision-making process seriously, and we were all relieved when all the patients were on schedule.

We were like three little kids hoping we wouldn't get caught with a hand in the cookie jar. The taste of "no toxicity" was sweet.

Third Week

One month beyond the autumnal equinox. Whether feeding the horses in the morning or coming home in less light, too late for an evening ride, I could feel the increasing darkness.

Driving into NIH on this third week in October, I noticed that the bright colors of September had fallen to the ground and were turning brown.

A good-news Board greeted me. Robert "Gosh" Thurman and Billy "Bear" Sullivan, my two luminaries of this week, would brighten my day. Robert would probably have named his puppy, and Billy would want me to examine Bear.

Robert's opening salvo was "Sparky!"

"Good name," I said as Robert handed me a photo.

Billy greeted me with Bear, and my exam indicated his teddy was in good health.

By half past eleven, there was good news for both boys. While their white blood counts were low, they weren't dangerously low, so POMP could be started Monday afternoon.

• • •

Every Tuesday morning, I examined Monday's bone marrow aspiration site. Immediately after removing the aspiration needle, the nurse pressed a sterile gauze sponge on the puncture site to stop any bleeding. After a minute, she placed a Band-Aid over the wound. On

Tuesday morning, I'd ask the patient to roll over and examine the aspiration site.

On this Tuesday morning, Billy was quiet. He rolled over as requested. No observable problems. After I replaced the old Band-Aid with a new one, Billy pointed to Bear's backside to indicate he wanted one for Bear.

Mrs. Sullivan finally said, "I'm afraid the bone-marrow aspirations are getting to Billy."

"I'm not surprised."

After a deep sigh, she told me of an incident when Billy had asked her for a pin while she was sewing. She gave him a large hatpin. Billy then turned Bear over and proceeded to do a marrow on his teddy. "He was pretty aggressive with the pin, and the whole scene was a little disturbing."

"Aggressive with the pin." Unfortunately, there's no way to get marrow without being aggressive. Sitting back in my chair, I remembered a presentation of play therapy from my two months of pediatrics as a junior medical student. Playing with dolls, children can demonstrate how they feel. Give a little boy from a family of four dolls—a daddy, a mommy, a little sister, and a brother—and ask him to tell a story. If he throws the daddy doll away and says, "I don't need him," you've learned something.

"Did Billy tell you what Bear said or felt after the marrow?"

"No. But, Doctor Humphrey, after Billy pulled the hatpin out of Bear, he picked up Bear, held him next to his shoulder, and said, 'It's over, Bear; I carry you back.'"

• • •

When I passed out carrots that night, I was in a low mood. The bone-marrow aspirations were getting to me, too. Billy wasn't the only one who had trouble with Monday morning. The nurses had told me that they hated bringing a crying patient into the treatment room and then holding the child down.

I had suppressed my feelings because telling a mom that her son or daughter was still in remission was a professional and personal positive event. Still, it was the patient who paid for the good news.

• • •

After a slow Wednesday morning, I had one patient to see in the afternoon: my one outpatient case, Carl Shively, and his memorable mom. I had spontaneously given most of my patients nicknames, but nothing had come to me for Carl.

While waiting, I pondered what sort of handle would fit the youngster. Carl was hospitalized only once at diagnosis and thereafter had been on daily 6-MP. Carl "6-MP" Shively captured what made him unique, but it lacked color.

Carl "Long-Term" Shively reflected his three-year response to therapy but was dull. Then there was Carl's mother. She had been dealing with chemotherapy for over three years. I liked the way she supported her son. She was a strong woman, and so were her friends.

Wow. Where do they get mothers like this? Carl was lucky to be alive, lucky to have a mom like Mrs. Shively, and lucky to have friends who'd been through it all. That's it! He'll be Carl "Lucky" Shively or just "Lucky Carl."

"I'm sorry we're late, Doctor Humphrey," Mrs. Shively said. "Let's get this marrow over, and afterward I'll tell you why it took me so long to get organized today."

Carl's marrow was free of leukemia. There were three very happy people in the clinic.

"Two months ago when we drove over here from Alexandria, we talked and joked about who would be our next doctor. Silly jokes, like how many heads he would have, would he speak English—you know, that kind of stuff. We lucked out. You're OK, Doc. But this morning, all I could think about was leukemia. I'm generally scared when I have to cross the Potomac River. Today, the Key Bridge is almost too narrow for crossing."

• • •

S itting on my desk were my two friends, an English and a medical dictionary. For me, these two books were more important for spelling than word definition, and *placebo* wasn't in either.

Jerry and Rick were working at their desks. "How do you spell *placebo*?"

"P-l-a-c-e b-o," Jerry said with a frown. "It's got to be in one of those books!"

"Ah, here it is. Thanks, Jerry. When you try to spell it and you begin with *plec*, or *plic*, or *plis*, you can't find it. That's my dyslexia showing up."

Rick stopped reading and said, "Really!"

When Jerry said he didn't know too much about dyslexia, Rick explained that this condition occurred in 5 to 10 percent of kids. "It's an impairment of an individual's ability to understand written language— difficulty with spelling and reading."

When Jerry said it must be something a kid can outgrow, I said, "Not so; you just have to learn to outmaneuver this handicap. I'm still a slow reader. If in med school my nondyslexic classmates went to bed at ten o'clock, I went to bed at midnight."

Rick said, "As a pediatrician, I counsel parents. Tell us a bit about your childhood experience with dyslexia."

"I liked books, loved to be read to as a preschooler, and liked going to the library but picked out books with lots of pictures. My parents thought I'd do well in school. When my mother was told by my teachers that they were going to make me repeat the second grade, she demanded that they retest me in the fall. My mother tutored me in phonics and word recognition for the entire summer. In the fall, my scores were at the fourth-grade level."

"And you went on to college and med school," Jerry said.

"A family emphasis on education hung over my head. All my aunts and uncles were college graduates, and on my father's side of the family, college education went back three generations. There were no MDs in the family, but there were lots of teachers, PhDs, and professors."

"What helps you now?" Rick asked.

"A habit of admitting without embarrassment that I'm dyslexic is important. When asking for help, I explain the problem. If someone corrects me on a word, I always thank them and ask them to continue to correct mistakes. Phonics is generally a good tool for me. *Placebo* is a good example. If I now remember to mispronounce the word as *place-bo* in my head instead of *ple-se-bo*, I'll be able to write it."

"Weeell, now, Ben." We all knew each other well enough that this opening meant Jerry was going to break into a comedy routine. "The University of Chicago doesn't accept toooo many dummies into its graduate schools," Jerry said, slurring. "Don't you think o-n-e doctoral degree would have been enough to keep up the Humphrey family tradition? Don't you think two doctoral degrees and a postdoc year in a foreign country is overdoing it a bit?"

I laughed until tears came to my eyes. "You guys are great. In this office, it's no problem to bare one's soul. That's b-e-a-r w-o-n's s-o-l-e."

We all laughed.

Fourth Week

The days were dreary. Dawn and dusk closed in on each other, and the nostalgia of autumn was over. Stopping to buy gas on the way into NIH, I noticed the adjacent restaurant's windows were decorated in orange and black and a small plastic skeleton hung on the café door.

It should have been a good week. I didn't need to go to the Board to see who was coming in: the happy trio was to be admitted. My one-year-old,

Michelle "Snuggle Bunny" Karr, my ten-year-old, Tammy "Pied Beauty" Long, and finally, my dog-loving six-year-old, Todd "Ralph" Yardley.

Pulling into the parking lot at NIH, I looked forward to treating this trio for the next five days. That was before I looked at Monday morning's bone-marrow aspirates.

I was up in the path lab by a quarter to ten. Oh shit, I thought. Tammy Long's aspirate contained some very bothersome cells. Not a lot—two or three in most fields—but they were easy to find. These cells were called blasts, a sign of a relapse of leukemia.

John, my tutor and head of the path lab, joined me on the two-headed microscope. In a few seconds, John sighed. "Yeah, we've got to call 'em blasts. Did you do a cell count, Ben?"

"Yes, sir. Seven percent blasts."

John asked a tech to stain three more slides and pull Tammy's original marrow at diagnosis. "Sometimes the morphology of the blasts at diagnosis can help differentiate leukemia from regenerating normal cells." Then he added, "Sometimes you can't tell. That's why a marrow is counted as remission if there are less than five percent blasts."

We looked at Tammy's diagnostic marrow together and then again at today's aspirate.

"What do you think we're dealing with this morning?" John asked.

"Leukemia."

"That's right."

I called Freireich and told him we had a questionable marrow we wanted him to look at and then added, "Now—please."

While we waited, John did a count of a thousand cells and asked me to look for clusters of blasts on the other smears.

Jay looked up from the scope and asked John what percent he got.

"I got eight percent; Ben got seven percent."

"What do you want to do, Doctor Humphrey?" Jay asked.

Having had time to think while waiting for Jay, I had an answer. Twenty-five or more leukemia cells in the marrow was a protocol failure, and POMP was discontinued. "Give her another course of POMP."

"Do it," Jay said and left.

I had the presence of mind to thank John for his help and should have thanked Jay for coming up. "Well, John, I'll go talk to the mom and tell her there's been a partial relapse."

"Now you know why I'm a pathologist," John uttered in a low voice. "Looking at cells is one thing. You've gotta talk to a mother and her daughter."

Riding in the elevator down to 2 East, I realized I was in a Freireichian mode. Give her POMP. Who cares if she vomits? Getting rid of those god-damn cells was the first priority. I was willing to put Tammy at risk of a fatal toxic complication. I wasn't used to thinking this way.

The biggest problem wasn't a question. It was a vivid prediction that Tammy was going to die.

• • •

Michelle Karr was in remission. The nurses took turns holding her on their laps, and I got my turn while relating the good news to Mrs. Karr.

Planning on having a running IV on Michelle before lunch, I had spent at least sixty minutes trying to find a suitable vein. Most of the time had been spent looking, and none of my three attempts with the needle were successful. Rick said he'd be glad to try after lunch.

During lunch, I vented some of my frustration over all this IV thera-py. Both Rick and Jerry were sympathetic.

Jerry asked Rick about IV therapy during his fellowship in Minnesota.

Rick shrugged. "Most of the therapy was oral, except vincristine or Oncovin as we call it in the POMP protocol."

Oncovin could only be given intravenously, and the oral mainte-nance therapy wasn't surprising. Most of the recent chemotherapy trials published in the medical literature administrated 6-MP, methotrexate, and prednisone orally.

At a quarter past two in the afternoon, Rick walked into the office. "I'm sorry, Ben. I couldn't find a vein."

Good old Jerry said he'd be glad to try, but I told them both that I'd go see Freireich and try to work out an oral schedule.

As usual, Jay's door was open, and his secretary told me to go right in. I laid my case before Jay in rational terms and forgot about compassion. His denial was pragmatic, dispassionate, and absolute. "Even if you could get Michelle to swallow all of those drugs, she'd vomit."

"We could spread the administration of the drugs over the entire day and not give them all at one time."

"And when she does vomit, how are you going to know how much drug was absorbed?" Freireich said. "Repeating the dose might be too much, resulting in toxicity. Give her a reduced dose, and she might relapse."

He had me; we both knew it.

"You're always welcome to come here with problems," Freireich remarked, "but you knew I wasn't going to let you use oral therapy before you came up here, didn't you?"

"Yes, sir. But this way, I can tell Michelle's mom that we had this conversation."

"I don't mind being the bad guy," Jay asserted.

"No need to put it that way. Mrs. Karr is an intelligent woman; she'll understand accurate dosing of drugs."

"Well then, this was a valuable use of my time," Jay said. He looked at me and added, "And yours too."

Jerry walked into the office at 3:20 p.m. "I finally got an IV going on Michelle. It took two sticks. God, she looks like a pincushion."

• • •

Todd was the last of the trio to be admitted. I wanted to be animated about *Mary Poppins* but thought, Humphrey, you'd better do the marrow first. You don't want to be a clown at nine and then the grim reaper at eleven.

At 11:20 a.m., I burst through the door to Todd's room and exclaimed, "Supercalifragilisticexpialidocious, you're in remission." I was in a good mood. I couldn't help thinking, the good news is you're OK; the bad news is that means you get POMP.

After Mrs. Yardley gave Todd a hug, she turned to me and said, "I gather you saw the film."

"Well, as the song says, *supercalifragilisticexpialidocious* is what you say when the cat's got your tongue. No leukemia cells, so I needed a special word."

"We got Todd the record."

After I asked Todd if he could sing "A Spoonful of Sugar," he obliged. He got through the entire song in a variety of keys. Delightful.

I told Mrs. Yardley that it would be a blessing if we had a spoonful of sugar for each of the next five days.

"Well, Doctor Humphrey," Mrs. Yardley replied, "there are the nurses."

• • •

Frank decided to throw a Halloween party. We'd return to the joys of childhood, carve pumpkins, wear costumes, eat candy corn, and decorate the cabin. We'd also sing folk songs, each of us knowing people who liked folk music. Frank had his guitar, and I had my banjo.

Halloween fell on Saturday night. This was Frank's party, so most of the guests were his acquaintances. The party was a lot of fun. Some couples tried eating an apple hung from a string, others bobbed for apples, and there was a pumpkin-carving contest.

Folksinging got under way later. We started with songs that everybody knew: "Go Tell Aunt Rhody," "This Land Is Your Land," and "The Frozen Logger."

Breaking Little Bones

Frank suggested we sing the echo song, "Oh, You Can't Get to Heaven." Each of us was to take a turn singing a traditional verse or, better still, making up a new verse. He started out:

> Oh, you can't get to heaven
> (Oh, you can't get to heaven)
> On roller skates
> (On roller skates)
> 'Cause you'd roll right by
> ('Cause you'd roll right by)
> Those pearly gates
> (Those pearly gates)
>
> Oh, you can't get to heaven
> On roller skates
> 'Cause you'd roll right by
> Those pearly gates
> I ain't-ah gonna grieve my Lord no more

Everybody was in the spirit to sing. A few people sang traditional verses, but several made up amusing original material. When my turn came, I sang:

> Oh, you can't get to heaven
> (Oh, you can't get to heaven)
> On POMP therapy

Laughter from the NCI group. Someone chimed in, "But a lot of people do." Someone else wanted in on the joke, and it was explained that POMP was an antileukemic therapy that caused patients to vomit. "Come on, Ben, you need to finish the verse."

> Oh, you can't get to heaven
> (Oh, you can't get to heaven)

G. Bennett Humphrey

On POMP therapy
(On POMP therapy)
'Cause the Lord don't want
('Cause the Lord don't want)
No pukin' up there
(No pukin' up there)

Again some laughter. I didn't know it that evening, but it was going to be months before I would again feel comfortable turning POMP into a joke.

Part II: Regrets

NOVEMBER

First & Second week

On the first Tuesday of November, I drove into NIH in murky pre-dawn light. A partially cloudy sky revealed a crescent moon hanging above the eastern horizon. Much of the landscape was shrouded in dark-gray fog.

This morning 2 East was quiet and gloomy. No kids were moving about in the hall, the nurses were in report, and the doctors' office was empty.

I wanted to see each of my kids to review their status before rounds with Freireich. Rick and Jerry were soon on the floor, and each of us went about our tasks without conversation.

Freireich entered the office slowly, took a deep breath as he sat down, sighed, and dropped his shoulders. He addressed us by first name and, after our case presentations, thanked us—which was unusual. From our perspective, there was a lack of tension because all the kids were on schedule. At the conclusion of rounds, Jay informed us that Tom Frei wanted to see all three of us in his office on the twelfth floor. Something was up. We did not talk on the elevator, make jokes, or speculate. In Dr. Frei's office, he invited us to sit in a semicircle of chairs. He then took a fourth chair that faced us.

"Jay and I want to review with you our perspective on how things have been going on 2 East," he said in a neutral tone. "We both know you're clinically very competent, the nurses respect you, and mothers often tell the nurses they like the way you interact with their children: Rick, you talk about becoming a father; Jerry, your tall tales of Paul Bunyan are entertaining; and Ben, I understand you put puzzles together and talk about dogs."

All these details without reference to notes.

"Jay and I are very aware of the enormous stress in caring for kids suffering from toxicity. All deaths are difficult; the nurses have told me about a few that seem more memorable than others: Jennifer Johnson, Betty Miller, and Jimmy Paul. We know that 2 East could easily be staffed by two clinical associates, but we have three on the floor in an attempt to spread the stress out over three physicians rather than two."

No one spoke.

"Toxicity is always a problem. It is to your credit as human beings that you want to prevent suffering in children, but that emotional involvement with your patients has resulted in protocol violations that interfere with our research." His manner was smooth; he never suggested he was angry with us or even disappointed in our performance.

"Let's compare leukemia to tuberculosis. In the previous century, the world was full of TB sanatoriums. History books brimmed with the names of promising young people who died of this now-nonfatal infection. The disease was associated with coughing up blood, respiratory failure, and a slow, ugly death. It took time to learn which drugs to use and how to use them in combination. Jay and I are involved in the same process. We know which drugs to use, and we are now learning how to combine these agents."

"Jay and I want each of you to think about what you have been doing," Tom said, and then he laid out a specific plan. Each of us in turn would be relieved of all clinical responsibilities for two weeks. This would not be vacation time, nor were we to take vacation leave. We were to report to the information desk each morning; we should not ask anyone how this or that kid was doing. We could go to lectures, the library, or the laboratory that we would be working in next year. During these two weeks, the physician off duty was not to take call. Rick was to be off the first two weeks, Jerry the second, and I the last.

"Think about what you have done to a major research effort to cure leukemia. Think about your clinical responsibilities. I want you to recognize that you're here to help the research staff try to cure this disease."

Tom stood up and thanked us for coming to his office; we left in silence.

• • •

No one talked as we rode the elevator down to 2 East. I had no control over my thoughts or emotions. After working together for four months, the three of us were close enough for me to assume that Rick and Jerry were going through the same turmoil.

In the doctors' office, Rick started to tell me of the status of two patients I would be following. I realized my mind was not focused. "I need to write this down on a piece of paper."

Never had I experienced this type of internal confusion. I had interfered with someone else's research. I was trained in the discipline of research and wanted an academic career. The safety and appropriateness of POMP was reviewed by an external committee. What if the chance of seeing another Jennifer was one in a hundred thousand? I had always been reliable. What would the faculty at the U of C think? Maybe I ought to switch to another field of medicine, one that didn't require patient care.

Underlying these erratic thoughts were feelings of guilt and emptiness. My irrational mind and disturbed emotional state were both in overdrive, and my head and heart could not contain the discord.

That night at the fence, I was haunted by my first encounter with Doctor Eugene Goldwasser when I asked if he would be my PhD adviser. He had only one rule for working in his laboratory. "We all make mistakes. Never try to cover up a mistake. Just come and tell me what happened, and we'll find a way to take care of the problem."

That was how I had been raised. My father had also made it clear that owning up to mistakes was the best way to handle things.

Our toxicity-reduction plan wasn't a mistake. What we had done— no, what *I* had done on 2 East was intentional, deliberate, and planned.

• • •

During our formal presentations on rounds, Jay never directly or indirectly reminded us of our protocol violations. He might have been disappointed with our performance, might have been angry that we had interfered with the research, might have felt that we had been immature, but I never detected these reactions, never felt my nose being rubbed in it.

Thinking back to that morning in Frei's office, the decision to have him talk to the three of us was well conceived. Tom was a distant figure, the internist on 12 East and coauthor of the POMP protocol. The three of us were close to Jay, knew some of his modus operandi. While we might not have been comfortable confronting him, we were not afraid to challenge him. If Jay had told us we were out of line, we might have reacted differently, but the outcome would have been the same. I never ceased to marvel at the multiple and very effective personae Jay could bring to bear. I had no idea then and still don't know what Jay told Dee and the other nurses. They continued to assist us in the same manner, going out of their way to be helpful. One might say they covertly supported us, just as they overtly cared for our kids.

• • •

"Do you know where Doctor Sandler is, Doctor H.?" Morgan asked. "We have an emergency admission coming in, and he's on call."

It was 4:50 p.m. Jerry had gone home at 4:30 p.m., so I told Morgan I'd be glad to take the case.

Morgan held a small piece of paper, looked at it, and read, "It's an eleven-year-old boy, Jeff Donaldson, who has the superior vena cava syndrome." She looked up. "I've never seen a child with that diagnosis."

"Neither have I, but I've read about it because the syndrome is an emergency. Doctor Freireich should be notified."

"He called the information to the floor, Doctor Humphrey."

"Jeff might need a tracheotomy."

"He already has one."

"Then, he's a full-blown emergency, and he's gonna need radiation therapy and low-dose steroids." Picking up the phone, I called radiotherapy and was told Freireich had already called and someone would be here shortly.

I pulled a folder from my desk labeled "Superior Mediastinal Syndrome / Superior Vena Cava Syndrome."

I told Morgan we could talk about the syndrome while waiting for Jeff. Not wanting to insult her knowledge, I parenthetically commented on the meaning of terms that were not commonly used in pediatrics. Lymphomas—or lymphosarcomas as they are sometimes called—are masses of cancerous white cells that can occur in the superior mediastinum, or upper chest. They grow rapidly, block venous return from the head, causing edema and plethora—flush or dusky appearance due to extra blood—in facial tissues, and can sometimes even obstruct the venous return from the arms. The tumors can narrow the trachea or cause tracheal deviations that result in a cough or dyspnea—difficulty breathing. The chest x-ray might demonstrate a pleural effusion, and the patient should not lie down because of orthopnea—respiratory distress in the supine position. There is a very high death rate at diagnosis, and medical procedures should be kept to a minimum; tracheotomy should be done in the sitting position.

We were about to discuss the clinical presentation and the high incidence of conversion to leukemia when the phone rang.

Barbara answered it. "Jeff's on his way up."

Two men came down the hall pushing a gurney with the back support raised. Jeff was sitting up, and a green oxygen tank lay next to his thighs with the tubing connected to a face mask strapped over the trach. At the foot of the gurney were a chest x-ray, several handwritten notes on hospital stationery, and laboratory slips.

The articles in my file contained several photos of kids with the syndrome, reproductions of chest x-rays with narrowed and displaced trachea, and clinical descriptions of the respiratory distress, but none of it prepared me for Jeff. Yes, his neck was swollen, yes, there was facial edema and a dusky color to his cheeks, and yes, he was sitting up, but it was the look of panic that most struck me. His eyes were fixed as if paralyzed and his mouth slightly open as if he had just witnessed some horrific crime. Jeff was terrified, and the only thing he could focus on was trying to breathe.

Without thinking, I donned the persona of a physician treating an emergency: *A*, airway—he's got one; *B*, breathing—he's still doing that. "Get some humidified oxygen going, and get the crash cart down here," I said. *C*, cardiac status—I listened to his heart for a few seconds— tachycardia—not surprising. While my stethoscope was out, I listened to his chest—no breath sounds on the lower right side; *D*, drugs—or in Jeff's case, hydrocortisone and radiation therapy. I guessed at his hydration status by feeling his forearm only to notice a few dilated veins. Dammit, there was compromised venous return of the upper extremities; the IV would have to go into a foot. He was dehydrated, which was no surprise; with that neck, he probably hadn't wanted to take time from breathing to drink anything. "Get an IV tray, lab slips for CBC, chemistries, and peripheral blood smear, please."

By now the nursing staff had joined us in the hall. "Do you want us to weigh him?" someone asked.

"No," I replied, trying to project calm with my voice. "I don't want him moved any more than necessary. He's probably thirty-five to forty kilos, and we'll assume he's one meter square."

Breaking Little Bones

"You can keep him on our gurney until you're ready to transfer him to a bed," an ambulance attendant volunteered.

"We'll be glad to hang around and help move him," the other attendant added.

Thanking them, I picked up the chest x-ray from the gurney and held it up to the overhead light. It was all there, just like in the articles: tracheal deviation, narrowing above the trach tube, and right pleural effusion.

Putting the x-ray down, I found myself face-to-face with Jay Freireich. I handed him the chest x-ray.

Jay put his hand on Jeff's shoulder and said, "I know you're frightened. We're going to give you some medicine to make it easier for you to breathe."

"I'm glad to see you." I finally took time for a deep breath and a sigh. In a rapid exchange of four or five comments, we reviewed a plan: IV and blood work first, hydrocortisone second, start IV fluids for rehydration, and then down to radiation therapy.

Within ten minutes we were on our way to radiation, the two ambulance attendants pushing the gurney and opening doors while Morgan held Jeff's hand, reassuring him. I pushed the larger oxygen tank, and Jay brought up the rear holding the x-ray and reading the handwritten notes from the referring hospital in Maryland.

Thirty-five minutes later we were back on the ward. The two guys carefully lifted Jeff onto his hospital bed with its head raised so he would be in a sitting position.

Morgan volunteered to stay with Jeff. Jay thanked the two attendants for all their help.

"Anytime. We hope he's better tomorrow."

I went to Jeff's room with his chart. I needed to sign off on the verbal orders that the nurses had recorded and write more formal admitting orders. Time to sit down and recognize I was nervous and coming down from an adrenaline high.

I went over to Jeff. His mouth was closed, the terrified stare in his eyes had softened, and his head was resting on his pillow. Morgan was standing at the bedside. She handed me a graphic display of Jeff's vital signs showing heart rate and respiratory rate were less rapid. I asked if she would like me to get a stool from the treatment room. She nodded, so I fetched one.

Returning to the doctors' office, I put my file on superior vena cava / superior mediastinal syndrome onto my desk. Thank God—John Graham with his abdominal lymphoma had inspired me to look into the literature on lymphomas.

After a quick meal in the cafeteria, I returned to Jeff's room at 6:40 p.m. Barbara was at the bedside. Jeff was awake, and Barbara told me he was dozing off for short periods but that he woke startled.

I called Jay at home and told him there was some good news. After reviewing Jeff's status, Jay said he appreciated the call. "Well, I so often bring you bad news; I thought it might be nice to share some good news."

I hung around for awhile and then remembered my kids on the floor. I made social rounds, listening to Sally Carter, chatting with Robert Thurman, and having one final look at Jeff.

On the way home, I thought of that first day when Billingsworth pointed to a stack of charts and commented that all the pertinent information was on the pillowcases. But kids don't have to bleed on their pillow like Billy Sullivan, or vomit breakfast like Sarah Thompkins, or produce bile-stain emesis like John Graham.

Pillows are for resting, and Jeff was alive, busy using his.

• • •

Early the next morning, I walked into Jeff's room at a quarter past seven to find Dee wiping his face with a wet washcloth and Brigid holding his hand, telling him he was OK.

Dee said, "He's a little upset but OK. We just drew the seven o'clock blood studies you ordered."

Brigid handed me the overnight graph of vital signs. There was further decline in both respiratory and heart rate, but both were still elevated.

After I said good morning to Jeff, I examined the tracheotomy site—no signs of bleeding; listened to his chest—no change there; looked at the IV site in the foot—no swelling; palpated his abdomen—no enlargement of the spleen or liver. His skin felt like there had been improvement in the turgor, and I wanted to believe there was less distension of the veins in his arms.

In the nurses' station, I reviewed the vital signs on Sally Carter, Robert Thurman, and two of Rick's kids who were also my responsibility. All four were on monthly POMP, all were on schedule, only one was nauseated or vomiting, and all were afebrile. That would be the last good patient news of the day.

Jerry hit the floor at 7:20 a.m. He hadn't had breakfast either and suggested we go together after he checked on his kids.

Before we went down to the cafeteria, I showed him Jeff's chest x-ray. His first reaction was one of dismay, and then he commented that he was supposed to take any new admissions. I just shook my head and waved the remark away. "That's the last thing the two of us need to worry about." Over breakfast, we discussed Jeff's problem, and later I gave him my file on the superior vena cava syndrome.

John from pathology called me at half past eight to tell me he had received a package from a hospital in Maryland on an eleven-year-old named Jeffrey Donaldson. The package contained some slides of a biopsy obtained when a tracheotomy had been performed, the tissue blocks, peripheral blood smears, laboratory reports, and a summary of an emergency-room visit.

In the path lab, I described Jeff's clinical presentation. We sat down at one of the double-headed microscopes, and John showed me the lymphosarcoma infiltration in the biopsy. "I gather the anesthesiologist insisted on using local rather than general anesthetic and also that the trach be done in the sitting position," John remarked. "He's a smart cookie, and they're lucky this kid didn't die on them." John went on to say, any unnecessary motion and requiring the patient to lie down will increase the already compromised venous return and can cause a cardiac arrest. If you use a general anesthetic on these kids, or make 'em lie down, spend time doing a lot of x-rays, you'll kill 'em for sure."

"About half of these young boys —the syndrome is more common in boys—will have a leukemic conversion during the course of their illness," John explained. The peripheral blood smear from the referring hospital was "clean, no leukemia cells."

I told him that last night's and this morning's CBC suggested that the bone marrow was functioning and handed him Jeff's chest x-ray.

John's normal view of a patient was a bone-marrow aspirate, or a peripheral blood smear. But in this case, he walked over to a viewing box and looked at the film. "So this is what life has handed an eleven-year-old," he said slowly.

I was about to learn that life had handed Jeff a whole lot more than just respiratory distress. There were a number of photocopies of notes and lab slips included with the tissue sections. The anesthesiologist's note stopped me dead in my tracks: "Jeff Donaldson is an eleven-year-old boy admitted in acute respiratory distress from the Margaret Aldrich Orphanage…"

An orphan! Last night I was so preoccupied with his respiratory distress I hadn't asked to speak to his mother. This morning my focus was on his clinical status. I hadn't asked if she had come in yet. There wasn't going to be a mother. The nurses were the ones who not only watched over him and recorded his vital signs but also held his hand, used a cool, wet washcloth to wipe his face, and told him things were OK.

I got on the phone and asked social services to get me as much information as possible on Jeff from the orphanage.

Was there anybody for Jeff, or was he all alone at eleven?

• • •

At 2:20 p.m., a Mrs. Linda Holmquist from social services entered our office on 2 East. She was probably forty, wearing a black-and-red plaid jacket and matching skirt, her light-brown hair streaked with white. When referring to her notes, she wore clear plastic reading glasses with rectangular lenses. Initially, her presentation of Jeff's record was factual. "This is a sad story about Jeff," she said.

Nodding, I said, "I agree."

"Just wait," she said. "Apparently Jeff was abandoned as an infant; no one knew what his real name was or his official birth date. There was one bright spot in Jeff's life. He had been taken into the home of a childless elderly couple as a foster child. They gave him the name of Jeff, and allowed him to be registered under their family name, and set his birthday as the twenty-first of March. It must have been a loving home," she said and started to cry.

After giving her a box of tissues, I said, "We all feel the same way, Mrs. Holmquist."

She wiped a few tears away and continued, "I don't even know this child." She paused and repeated, "It must have been a very loving home. Jeff did very well at school; he'd been given music lessons—I think the clarinet—and because of their age, Jeff referred to them as Granddad and Grandma. Then, when Jeff was ten, Granddad Donaldson died, and some official decided that Grandma was too old and weak to care for Jeff. She was admitted to some sort of facility for the elderly, and Jeff went to the orphanage." Mrs. Holmquist straightened up, blew her nose, and concluded, "Jeff has not made any friends at the orphanage, and he no longer cares about school." There was a long pause, and finally she said, "They didn't even ask how he was doing."

"Let's call the orphanage and—"

"Don't bother," she said. "In all fairness, Doctor Humphrey, they're short of staff, underfunded, have big budget problems. Just feeding the kids is a problem." She paused. "The orphanage will send one set of clothes for Jeff and also a few personal things, things he's fond of. I guess there's no one for Jeff."

"Well, I know four nurses who are already very involved; he's now in very good hands." I was almost in tears. "Very caring hands."

• • •

That evening, I pondered what was going on in my professional life. For the last two weeks, I'd been working with Jerry. For the next two weeks, I'd be working with Rick, and for two weeks after that, I wouldn't be on 2 East. That would be mid-December, and then there would be two weeks until Christmas and the New Year. Life was now showing up in two-week intervals.

On Saturday at 8:20 a.m., I wrote an order in Jeff's chart: "Change clinical status from Critical to Stable." The official path report was back, so I also changed the admitting diagnosis from tumor to lymphoma and in my progress note wrote, "Superior mediastinum syndrome responding to radiation therapy and hydrocortisone."

At 12:10 p.m., Morgan was at Jeff's side helping him with lunch. Not wanting to interrupt, I told Morgan that this was just a social call. Even an internist knew that nutrition was important for a kid like Jeff, but there was a hell of a lot more going on than the intake of calories.

Both of Jeff's hands were free as the IV was in his foot, and I guessed that he could have fed himself but was obviously enjoying the interaction with his lunch companion. Morgan had broken a soft meat patty into bite-size pieces. Jeff would take, chew, swallow, and then look at her for approval. She would smile and nod. The exchange of affection was wonderful to behold. Jeff also liked the mashed potatoes. He was holding a fork and Morgan a spoon. After every fourth bite of potatoes or meat, she offered Jeff the tray's vegetable. Jeff opened his mouth for a spoonful of spinach.

I had to swallow a few unshed tears. Not because a kid had just died or relapsed but because Morgan was feeding Jeff and both were enjoying the moment.

Third and Fourth Week

Jerry's forced leave from 2 East started today.

Rick was on the floor before I arrived at a quarter past seven. He greeted me with that wonderful smile of his. We shook hands.

"Good to see you. How's Jody?"

After getting out the summary of the past two weeks, I explained that Jerry and I had made rounds together on all kids on the ward, and we agreed to continue that practice.

There was something different about working with this pediatrician. Rick was less direct about obtaining information from a mom. He waited for them to provide it. If something important needed to be ascertained, Rick had different ways of encouraging the mom to report a sign or symptom. For example, Jerry and I would ask if there were any bruises, but Rick was more likely to ask if the mother had noticed anything on the skin while dressing or bathing her son or daughter. The answer to Rick's question might reveal petechiae, but the answer to the question posed by Jerry or me might be no. There was something gentle and patient about Rick's manner and language. I enjoyed listening to him talk to a mom and watching him examine a child.

I wondered if that was a general attribute of pediatricians or whether Rick was a different kind of doctor, or better trained in wearing the persona of a physician, or just a warm human being who happened to be a doctor.

• • •

"Doctor Humphrey, there's a package from the Margaret Aldrich Orphanage that just arrived," Dee said. "It's a change of clothes for Jeff and what I assume are some of his personal things. We'd better make a list of what's in here."

G. Bennett Humphrey

In her office we opened a cotton bag about the size of a sheet of paper that closed with a drawstring. "Jeff" was written on the bottom. Dee opened it and removed the contents: ten green plastic vintage World War II soldiers, each two inches tall in various action poses; a Boy Scouts of America manual; a Cub Scout Bobcat pin; a small plastic collar, the size for a cat or small dog; and an envelope containing black-and-white photos.

While Dee noted the contents, I looked at the photographs.

"There are twenty-one, all black-and-white. The collar belonged to a cat." There was one photo of Jeff holding a kitten, another of Jeff holding a cat, and a family photo of Jeff, the cat, and an elderly couple. There were pictures of a childhood: a picture of Jeff probably taken when he was eight or nine in a band uniform, a clarinet in his mouth; another of Jeff standing very straight and tall in a Cub Scout uniform, his right hand at shoulder level, index and middle fingers raised. There were other photos of Jeff with one or both foster parents, photos of a small one-story frame house, photos from both Christmas and birthday parties, and one of Jeff as a baby in Grandma's arms in front of a church.

Dee looked through the pictures while I returned the rest of Jeff's personal items to the bag. "I'll go see Jeff."

Brigid and Jeff were working with a pad of paper, apparently drawing. Jeff sat up when he saw the bag, and I took each item out one at a time, placing it before him on his bedside table.

"May I look at the photos, Jeff?" Brigid asked.

No response. She looked through the collection, occasionally showing Jeff a photo and telling him, "That's a nice picture."

Jeff arranged the plastic soldiers in two groups. She handed him the photos. "You can keep these here in your room." She added, "Or we can store them at the nurses' station for safekeeping, and we'll bring them to you anytime you want."

Jeff returned the photos to their envelope and pushed them toward her. Everything else was returned to the bag except the soldiers.

When I asked, "Did Granddad and Grandma give you the soldiers?" he raised his head, almost smiled, and then nodded.

That was our first exchange, and it was over something important.

• • •

Rick asked me to use an ophthalmoscope to look at the optic nerves in one of his kids who was complaining of headaches. Because meningeal leukemia presented with headaches, Rick wanted to know if the optic nerve was normal. Rick introduced me to Mark and his mother, explaining that we were going to look into Mark's eyes. Neither of us saw any swelling or bulge of the optic nerve.

After saying he didn't find any abnormalities, Rick turned the ophthalmoscope around and let Mark look into his eye. For a few minutes, Mark forgot his headache. What a neat trick—something for me to do with Robert "Gosh" Thurman.

Rick had obviously discussed this problem with other mothers. "Mark, you've received intravenous methotrexate and 6-MP. These drugs leave the bloodstream and diffuse into the liver, spleen, lymph nodes, and other tissues of the body. The leukemic cells in these organs are killed by the drugs. But when your blood flowed through your brain, these drugs could not get into brain tissue. There's a barrier, a blood-brain barrier that protects your brain. The problem is that leukemic cells can cross that barrier and hide from the drugs. When that happens, the leukemic cells can get into the membranes of the brain, which are called the meninges, thus the name meningeal leukemia. These leukemic cells irritated the meninges and caused headaches." Rick said he'd be back to explain what was going to happen next.

Out in the hall, Rick said, "You know, I'm surprised we haven't had a case of meningeal leukemia before now. Steroids can cross the blood-brain barrier, and the high doses of prednisolone in POMP may be delaying the onset or decreasing the incidence of meningeal leukemia. Let's go talk to Freireich."

Jay listened to the case and said intraspinal methotrexate was at present the treatment of choice. "It's like we have two separate populations of leukemic cells to treat—you might even say two separate patients to treat."

Before we left, Jay observed that the testes, like the brain, were also lipid-rich organs and that testicular infiltration with enlargement was occasionally being reported now that remissions were lasting longer.

Was the future of research in leukemia just going to be one goddamn headache after another?

• • •

Jeff Donaldson was doing well. I brought the serial chest x-rays for Jay to review. The trachea was now in the normal position, and most of the pleural fluid had been reabsorbed. Jeff's neck appeared normal. I had asked for an opinion about removing the tracheal tube and closing the tracheotomy site. "Anytime," the surgeon from ENT remarked.

"Good idea. Get rid of that tube," Jay commented. "It's a foreign body, a focus for infection, and he needs to start on POMP; there's the high rate of leukemic conversions in kids with lymphomas of the neck." By conversion, Jay meant that the malignant cells that had been a solid mass or lymphoma were in some way transformed into individual circulating leukemic cells. In the older medical literature, leukemia was sometimes referred to as a liquid tumor.

In addition to the positive changes in Jeff's medical status, his face was now back to normal. He was a handsome young man.

"We're all jealous of his hair," Morgan said. "When the sunlight strikes his head, there's a golden hue to that crown. We love to wash, dry, and comb it."

"Yes. There's an angelic quality to his face." Then I added, "But *angelic* is not an adjective a preadolescent boy would appreciate."

"That's true," she said, "but Jeff's manner is so gentle, and he has a way of smiling to show his appreciation. I'll just think of him as my private angel."

"I like your description of his manner. He'll be 'Gentle Jeff.'"

The surgeon from ENT said they'd put Jeff on the OR schedule for the next day. This time it would be safe to use a general anesthetic. I told Jeff what I thought was the good news. After I explained general anesthetic to him, he frowned, shook his head, and leaned toward Morgan.

"Will you stay with Jeff for a few minutes, Doctor Humphrey?"

She returned and explained to me that Dee had said she could accompany Jeff up to the surgical suite. "I'll go with you up to the operating room. They're going to put you to sleep so you won't feel any pain, and when you wake up in the recovery room, I'll be there, Jeff."

Wow! Morgan had the insight to recognize that Jeff might not have liked breathing through a tube in his neck but that it was now part of his routine and 2 East was a safe place. Going to surgery threatened that routine.

I wondered if they taught that kind of stuff in nursing school. Or was it the children that brought out the best in all of us?

• • •

"**D**octor Humphrey, I know how you—we all hate restarting IVs, but physical therapy asked if we could transfer Jeff's IV to one of his hands so the IV in the foot could be removed. Then we can get him on his feet and help him regain his strength. But it's your decision, of course," Morgan said.

"Brilliant," I said.

A slight drop in her shoulders hinted that Morgan had been anxious about making the suggestion.

"Morgan, anytime you have an idea for helping these kids, our kids, please don't hesitate to bring it to my attention."

She smiled, thanked me, and left.

When I knocked on her door, Dee asked me to come in. After telling her about transferring Jeff's IV, I explained in polite terms that there was no room on 2 East for the traditional hierarchical relationship between the nurses and me as a physician.

Dee smiled, pushing back a pile of papers. "Doctor Humphrey, we have noticed that all three of you are open to and grateful for any suggestions we can make." She shook her head. "It's not always that way. Some years, it's like walking on pins and needles around here."

• • •

"Jeff has become what we refer to as 'the Child of the Floor,'" Dee said as she saw me studying the Board.

"A what?"

"A 'Child of the Floor' occurs when the mothers of 2 East unite in a common front to support one specific kid. Remember Betty Miller? One mother would sit with Betty while another took Mrs. Miller down to the cafeteria for coffee or a meal. Well, now Jeff is getting that extra maternal support. When my staff is busy with hanging chemotherapy infusion bags in the morning, there's a mother in Jeff's room, even if he's asleep."

But there was more to it than just babysitting. The nurses knew that I would restart Jeff's IV and must have mentioned it to one of the mothers. Mrs. Thurman and Robert visited Jeff. "An IV in your hand's better. You can walk around. You don't have to sit in a wheelchair," Robert said to Jeff.

There were other examples. Jeff didn't have any shoes. Mrs. Taylor, one of Rick's mothers, had a friend that owned a shoe store and would donate a pair of shoes. Another mom wanted to get Jeff some clothes, not secondhand but new clothes that fit and colors that matched.

After I told Rick about this surrogate-mother program, we went for coffee. Passing through the waiting room, we noticed three mothers sitting on the edge of the long couch exchanging ideas.

The therapeutic couch was now a command post.

• • •

Just prior to Thanksgiving, all of us began preparing Jeff for discharge. Physical therapy had helped Jeff regain his strength. Mrs. Holmquist visited Jeff and told him about a family that wanted him to stay with them for a few weeks. The Wagner family had a son two years younger than Jeff and a daughter his age. Jeff wasn't overjoyed at leaving 2 East. Mrs. Holmquist said he'd have a few days to get used to the idea and she'd personally introduce him to the Wagners.

By now, the surrogate mothers had assembled two changes of clothes and a pair of shoes. On Tuesday, Morgan and I went to see Jeff. She was carrying one change of clothes and his new shoes.

"Jeff, you're all done with those drugs that upset your stomach. You can leave the hospital on Thursday," I said.

Jeff looked at me as if he were a puppy I had just scolded. I felt terrible. It must have been written all over my face, because Morgan stepped forward and gave Jeff a gentle hug.

"That's good news, Jeff," she said. "It'll be good for you to get out of here for awhile. You can always come back, and we'll be happy to see you. Come on. Let's try on your new clothes."

I left Jeff in Morgan's capable hands.

When they came out, they were walking hand in hand, Morgan smiling fondly at Jeff as he skipped along beside her. "Show Doctor Humphrey your new shoes."

Jeff proudly put one foot forward and then the other.

"Are those good running shoes?" I asked.

At that Jeff trotted down to the end of the hall, turned, and ran back toward us.

"He liked his new clothes," Morgan said, "but when we put on his shoes, he lit up like a Christmas tree."

Jeff was happy in this moment, and Morgan and I could watch him as a happy friend. But his prognosis was grave, and I was reminded of the poem, *With Rue My Heart Is Laden.*

"He's now a 'light-footed lad.'"

"That's a nice description."

"It's not original, Morgan. I stole it from a poet named A. E. Housman."

• • •

When I arrived at Kirkhill, I looked for Housman in an anthology. I liked his "When I Was One-and-Twenty," but I didn't bother to read it. Rather I turned to another favorite poem:

> With rue my heart is laden
> For golden friends I had,
> For many a roe-lipt maiden
> And many a lightfoot lad.
>
> By brooks too broad for leaping
> The lightfoot boys are laid;
> The rose-lipt girls are sleeping
> In fields where roses fade.

I liked this poem because it flowed: *laden* rhymed with *maiden* and *had* with *lad*. It had added *rue* to my vocabulary. But tonight, I read it for the first time with a laden heart. I realized that, prior to 2 East, I'd not had any laden experience with death. When my grandparents died, my parents had spent time explaining that death of our elders was "the natural order of things." None of my peers in school had died; even as a medical student, none of my patients had died. As an intern and resident, I had experienced the death of adults. As a resident, the advice offered to me and the quality exhibited by my role models was "objectivity." On 2 East, objectivity wasn't working. It all too often left me with an emotional void, a sense that I didn't have the right or need to grieve.

We were out of carrots, so I got a flashlight, went to the barn and put a scoop of molasses and oats in each of three buckets. As I listened to the nickering, stamping of feet, and munching of feed, I concluded that one fact was haunting me: kids with lymphoma don't respond well to POMP. Jeff was likely to die, and so was John Graham.

• • •

"Will you take care of the animals for a few days?" Frank asked. "I want to go home to spend some time with my mom. Since my dad's death, holidays are lonely for her."

"Be glad to. Besides, I'm not going anywhere."

November had been a dreary month, in terms of both internal and external weather. I hadn't called or written my parents; there wasn't anything I wanted to share with them. I went about my tasks on 2 East without thinking. My routine POMP kids were all doing well.

On this day, Jeff walked off the floor wearing a matching outfit of a wool sweater, slacks, and light jacket. Mrs. Holmquist and Brigid accompanied him to the front door to meet the Wagners.

When I went through the cafeteria line for my lunch, I noted cranberry sauce and then the turkey in gelatinous gravy. That's right. Thanksgiving.

That afternoon, I wrote out my orders for the anticipated discharges the next day, reviewed everyone's vital signs again, and made social rounds. One of Jerry's moms said she hoped Doctor Sandler was enjoying Thanksgiving with his family. Because of his absence, she assumed he was back in Maine. I said something neutral, like that was what Thanksgiving was all about. I should have remarked that there was much to be thankful for as her son was in remission and doing well. But I didn't, and I felt bad that the thought hadn't come to me while I was in the room.

I had another Thanksgiving plate for dinner in the cafeteria. The place was almost deserted. The gravy was tasteless, the cranberries were in a jelly, not a whole-berry sauce, and the stuffing lacked the taste of sage and parsley. But the kitchen staff had tried. There were a few decorations of turkeys, pilgrims, and harvest scenes on the wall. I decided it was a good meal and went back into the kitchen to thank someone who looked like a chef.

• • •

Back at Kirkhill, I fed Shonto an extra helping of canned dog food, got out my collection of songs from the Old Town School of Folk Music, and read the second and third verses from "Trouble in Mind":

> *I'm all alone at midnight,*
> *and my lamp is burning low,*
> *Never had so much*
> *Trouble in my life before.*
>
> *I'm gonna lay my head*
> *On that lonesome railroad line,*
> *Let the Two Nineteen*
> *Pacify my mind.*

Well, Humphrey, you've got the blues. Don't indulge too deeply.

A cold wind out of the north caused me to shiver as I left the cabin. At the fence, my mind drifted back to childhood. At Thanksgiving, I'd hang around the kitchen for those magic aromas of cooked onions, advise my mother on how much more sugar was necessary for the cranberry sauce, and listen to her gentle voice tell how she learned to make stuffing from her own mother: a pinch of sage, a handful of parsley, chopped celery, and lots of onions, butter, and dried bread.

By the time the carrots were all gone, I was remembering the Thanksgivings of my graduate-student days when I would retreat to home and a morning of pheasant hunting. My parents' much-beloved golden retriever, Nugget, was from a long line of champions, and once a year her inherent skills dominated every fiber of her being. On Thanksgiving, Nugget was a prima ballerina, center stage. Instinctively, she knew how to work the field in a pas seul, and my father would say, "Who needs to attend the ballet?"

Childhood, home, family, graduate studies, and pheasant hunting all seemed long ago and far away.

DECEMBER

First and Second Week

Rick and Jerry would now be on 2 East while I was off. It felt like solitary confinement. I missed not doing puzzles or listening to my kids tell me about their world. I missed the feeling of awe and respect that so often occurred when I witnessed the extraordinary love shown by mothers toward their children. I missed seeing the nurses go about their day, at the bedsides providing care.

To my surprise, I didn't run to the laboratory and immerse myself in lab research. Despite my previous love of the library, now I went but learned little. Lectures in molecular biology seemed meaningless. During these two weeks, I wanted to be alone. During the day, I often took long walks around the NIH campus. At Kirkhill, I exchanged a few words with Frank, but much of the time he was gone. On the second weekend, I got out my copy of Remarque's *All Quiet on the Western Front*. I looked for and found the section where the main character, Paul Bäumer, is on leave from the trenches and goes home and visits his family. While there were differences in Paul's experience and my situation, we had one thing in common. Paul missed his friends from the trenches, and I missed my comrades from 2 East. And we had one truly important difference. Paul recognized he had changed. I needed to recognize my own changes.

Paul fought in World War I. In the summer of 1964, I had evaded Vietnam, but during the last five months, I realized I was a soldier in another kind of war. *All Quiet on the Western Front* spoke to me. During

November and now in December, I walked or lunged or rode Whirley-Wee, but that didn't bring balance to my life. The first two weeks of December were the worst. Wherever I found myself, I wasn't there.

• • •

Early in December, Kristina wrote to tell me of her planned holiday activities in Germany. I liked baroque brass music, so she described in some detail a program at Saint Rochhuskapelle in Bingen. She planned to spend Christmas with her family in Freiburg, a beautiful city on the edge of the Black Forest.

What was I doing for the holidays? I had no plans. In fact, I wasn't doing anything at all. Kristina had taken the time to write a thoughtful holiday letter, and I wanted to do the same. A blue sheet of thin paper lay before me. Blank.

Finally, I wrote of the pleasant memories of our December together. The holiday season began on the fourth Sunday before Christmas, when the first candle of the Advent wreath or *Der Adventskranz* was lit. Last year, she had helped me pick out an *Adventskranz* for my parents; I had enjoyed her explanation of the children's *Adventskalender*. During the second week of December, members of the laboratory brought in cake and cookies; *stollen* was my favorite. I reminded Kristina of the evening my professor invited me over for dinner. Before we sat down for a Christmas feast, he lit the candles on the tree. I had never seen real candles flicker on a Christmas tree and was enchanted. Before we went to the dining room, the candles were blown out for safety. To close, I wrote about a cold December evening when we went to the Christmas market, *Weihnachtsmarkte*, and had a glass of *Glühwein*. So many memorable things filled the page, and I was deep in that other December. A December "nice to remember."

• • •

G. Bennett Humphrey

Time at the fence during the first two weeks of December was different from my time with the horses during the summer and fall when I would worry about a problem that would be resolved within a period of time. Did Todd "Ralph" Yardley have a viral infection? On Monday, if there was no growth, we'd stop his antibiotics and send him home to Ralph. How was smiling and waving Betty Miller going to do? In the summer and fall months, I could call 2 East and find out.

Now in a cold December wind, I was still worrying about my kids. How was Michelle "Snuggle Bunny" Karr doing? Was Robert "Gosh" Thurman finding his new puppy an adequate diversion from soccer? Was "Gentle" Jeff Donaldson enjoying being with the Wagner family?

One night I told Domino, "I'm now in a two-week state of limbo, and I don't like it. On 2 East, there are short periods of limbo. I aspirate marrow, and twenty minutes later, I look at it and know if I'm going to have to deal with a relapse. One of my kids spikes a fever; I do a blood culture, start IV antibiotics, and within two days know if I'm dealing with sepsis. But now, Domino, I don't know which of my kids are doing well and which have problems. Not being on 2 East and not knowing and not being able to find out is hell."

• • •

Too often, I returned to Tom's statement: "I want you to think about what you have done to a major research effort to cure leukemia," he'd said. He could have scolded us, threatened us, but instead he admonished us, required us to change—and that was far more effective. He was disappointed in our performance. Tom's remark would interrupt my reading in the library or break my train of thought in a seminar.

I pondered a series of thoughts and questions on a long walk with Whirley-Wee. Was my problem a moral issue? One has to be free to judge whether an act is moral or immoral. Was I free? As a commissioned officer in a military branch of the uniformed services, I had orders to follow.

Breaking Little Bones

The toxicity of POMP pushed Rick, Jerry, and me over the edge of what we could tolerate. Jay could, in some way, tolerate it, but we couldn't. Sometimes I wondered if the kids and their moms tolerated 2 East better than me—probably not.

"You know, Whirley-Wee, I've bonded with these kids; I love 'em. I could say that's the problem, but I don't think so. I even feel that deep down inside of Freireich is a commitment to these children. Maybe 2 East, the reality of leukemia, and Jay's attempt to cure this malignancy are beyond good and evil."

I looked at my horse. None of this made any sense. Presently, I didn't think a rational explanation would come to me. Validation for my action of delaying therapy didn't seem appropriate. Maybe I'd always have to live with this experience of 2 East.

• • •

Sunday morning, the second weekend in December, the sky was overcast, and a damp wind blew out of the north. After feeding the horses, I decided to walk the fence line. Many of the posts were old and the wood a bit rotten. While they were strong enough to stand and support barbed wire, I planned to bind any loose strands to the post with a loop of smooth wire. In a toolbox in the barn, I found a pair of lineman's pliers and a spool of wire.

The horses stood in a huddle of three to get some protection from the wind. Shonto kept me company, but I felt alone.

Halfway down the southern fence line, one of those random questions came to me. Why had Rick, Jerry, and I so easily adopted the toxicity-reduction plan? None of us were elated when a patient's chart was off the floor on Tuesday. All three of us were headed for academic careers that required research if you wanted to be promoted or have your contract renewed. We were trained to think, not feel. Teaching was all fine and well, but research was king.

By the time I reached the far end, I recalled my exposure to the dichotomy of thinking and feeling in my first undergraduate course in psychology. Our professor had been a graduate student during World War II, and his thesis was part of a larger study on what he called psychological preferences. He discussed four pairs of preferences or dichotomies, although I could only vividly remember one pair: thinking and feeling.

But POMP was a schedule to be followed, not a question of thinking or feeling when to start the next course. A dichotomy I'd have to live with.

By now, I was checking the western fence line that ran parallel to Route 28.

Jay Freireich was obviously a thinker. The POMP protocol was like a rule book. But Myron had told me, during our LD10 discussion of October that every week Jay would review the toxicity our kids were experiencing and ask the question, is POMP too toxic? Jay was willing to reduce the doses; that was his job.

Feeling was more common among women, but the nurses never whined about starting POMP. We never heard Morgan or Brigid ask, "Do we have to start today?" And all the nurses were just as involved with the kids of 2 East as we were—maybe more so. But they didn't have to write the orders.

I closed the gate, put the pliers and spool back in the toolbox, and returned to the fence. Humphrey, I thought, stop. Just get off it. Tomorrow you'll be back on 2 East. Your job is to write the POMP orders, the nurses will hang the infusion bags, and Jay will monitor toxicity.

Third and Fourth Week

Monday morning, and a drive back to the real world after a two-week void. We were together again, *Drie Kamaraden*. I still had horses, Jerry had Georgetown, and Rick had a pregnant wife. There was catching up to do, but first, all I wanted to know was the status of my kids.

"Ben, all of your kids on routine POMP did well, but I've got bad news about Tammy Long," Rick said. "We admitted her last week with bad bone pain. She presented last April with the same pain. Her mother knew it was a relapse before I even did the marrow."

"Oh boy. What a way to start the week," I muttered. "Is Tammy still on the floor?"

"No. Mrs. Long knew about daunomycin and wanted Tammy to receive a course. It did stop the pain, and we discharged her last Thursday."

"I'll call Mrs. Long."

"Ben, you've told me all about John Graham. He's still withdrawn, and I know you're concerned about his mother," Rick said.

"I'll also call Mrs. Graham," I sighed, not knowing exactly what I was going to say.

"You've got some really neat kids," Jerry said. "Sarah Thompkins didn't say a word all week long, but while Sally Carter was quiet on Monday, she started to talk on Tuesday, and she was talking as she walked off the floor on Friday. Good news—Jeff Donaldson is enjoying being with that family."

"Thanks, Jerry. That's great to hear, but you can't have either Sarah or Sally. I want 'em both back."

"Rick, how's your case of meningeal leukemia?" I asked.

"No more headaches. Intrathecal methotrexate seems to be working," Rick said.

"Thanks, guys. It's good to be back."

"Hi, Doctor H.," Morgan chirped. "Both Billy Sullivan and Robert Thurman are in good spirits, and their moms say they're OK." I examined Billy's Bear and looked at pictures of Robert's puppy, Sparky. There were bone marrows to do, but I was back in the groove. By 11:25 a.m. I had related to both moms that there were no bad cells.

I took a midday break and went to my bench to feed my buddy Squirrel, and tell him, "I'm back." I felt bad for not asking Rick or Jerry to feed him while I was gone.

Dee gave me the home number of the Grahams and the Longs. After getting the yellow pad of paper, I put it back. Humphrey, you don't have to organize what you're going to say. You know these moms, and they know you. After talking to the mothers, I spoke to each kid. "I'm glad the bone pain is gone, Doctor Humphrey," Tammy Long said. Then she added, "I'm going to have a good Christmas."

After John Graham got on the phone and said hello, I told him I was pleased his marrow had good cells. There was a pause, during which I overheard a maternal prompt, and John said, "Thank you, Doctor."

Hanging up, I sat back in my chair and reflected on a morning of good-news marrows and an afternoon of returning to reality.

• • •

On Tuesday morning after rounds with Jay, Billy Sullivan and I played with Bear. Mrs. Sullivan joined in the game using a monkey doll to ask questions of Bear.

At 11: 20 a.m. I went to see a new admission, Dan Martin, a five-year-old. "Our doctor said he thought Dan had leukemia," Mrs. Martin said. "But you'll be able to tell me what's really wrong with Dan," she quickly added. She patted her son on the thigh and took his hand.

Her statement suggested she was still hoping her son didn't have leukemia. I also wondered if their doctor had really said he "thought" it was leukemia. She was overtly nervous, hands shaking, drawn face with eyes red from crying. She held a handkerchief at the ready.

Back in August, Rick had said that one never guesses at the diagnosis of leukemia when talking to a mom. "You discuss differential diagnoses with medical students, not moms." Rick told me about a specific kid. "His mom had been told the anemia was probably iron deficiency. It was leukemia, but she spent a year questioning the diagnosis, wondering if her son shouldn't be given a trial of iron therapy, or why not check the iron level in the blood, and so forth."

So Mrs. Martin was going through the hell of "Could it really be leukemia?"

Dan was pale, a common enough sign of bone-marrow failure. He sat next to his mom, often looked up at her with a frown, and occasionally patted her forearm. Incredible, I thought. Here's a five-year-old doing the best he can to support his mother.

I tried to obtain the medical history, but Mrs. Martin didn't answer my questions: "Dan eats a balanced diet; no one in our family has ever had anything serious; his yearly checkup in August was fine."

No matter how I phrased my questions, I couldn't get a coherent history. I felt sorry for this mother and as if everything in my chest had sunk an inch or two. Finally, I realized that doing the marrow and getting a concrete diagnosis might be the best thing.

This mother needed to resolve her terrible state of uncertainty.

Up in the path lab, John Thomas and I looked at the marrow. No question about the diagnosis. We couldn't find a normal cell in the smears of Dan's marrow. I called Jay and asked him to come up. John frowned, and I explained that the mother was desperately trying to deny the diagnosis. "I'm young. Mrs. Martin may not know what a pathologist does, but I can explain to her that Jay has been diagnosing and treating leukemia for ten years," I said.

Jay looked up from the microscope. "ALL. I don't need the special stains to differentiate this one from AML." After John explained why I had asked for his opinion, Jay said, "You're using me again," and seeing me nod, he added, "Good use of my time."

It didn't help. On being told the diagnosis, Mrs. Martin's response was, "It can't be." I sat down again, trying to indicate there was no hurry. She wondered about this and that, and again I had that sinking feeling. I told her that Doctor Freireich had ten years of experience and had personally looked at Dan's marrow. She didn't want to meet him.

My next feeble attempt didn't work either. Going over to Dan, I told him, "Sorry about the pain of the marrow; we have drugs to make you feel better; we can start the treatment this afternoon; a blood transfusion will make you stronger." I included other things that I thought Mrs. Martin might want to hear, but she apparently ignored my comments to her son.

"Couldn't we wait a few weeks?" she asked.

I rang for the nurse, and Morgan came. After explaining that Mrs. Martin and Dan had just learned the diagnosis, I asked if she could stay in the room for a few minutes.

Trouble with a marrow, call Jay. Trouble with a mom, call an expert. I walked into Billy's room, where Mrs. Sullivan was reading to him. I asked if she would mind going to Dan's room to comfort Mrs. Martin.

"Of course. Of course!" Mrs. Sullivan said, tears flooding her eyes. She blew her nose. "I remember that first day. Oh God, I remember it well." She straightened up to her full height, wiped her eyes, set her shoulders, and explained to Billy she'd be back in a little while.

"Thanks, Mrs. Sullivan, he's in room five. I'll read the rest of the book to Billy. What page—"

She was out the door before I finished the sentence. At first, I had trouble concentrating. Billy knew the book so well that if I left a word out, he'd correct me. After making two or three mistakes, I created a different voice for each character and added sound effects.

Twenty minutes later, Mrs. Sullivan returned with both Mrs. Martin and Dan and said, "Billy, this is Dan. He wants to meet you."

• • •

"Lucky" Carl Shively's third outpatient visit was on Wednesday afternoon. Mrs. Shively gave me a concise history: Carl was doing well on his daily oral 6-mercaptopurine, and there were no signs or symptoms of relapse or toxicity. With her usual gusto, she told me that the pills were part of their daily routine, and Carl took it like candy. "We never miss a day." She babbled on about the central role of chemotherapy in their life and her gratitude for Carl's response to therapy.

Carl was Carl: no change, a cool kid. As usual, he had a comic book to read. Mrs. Shively said, "This is our fourth Christmas with Carl doing well."

It was a complete sentence but an incomplete thought. I knew that she would call her circle of friends—mothers from 2 East, mothers whose son or daughter had died. It was one thing to share Carl's good news any other time of the year, but at Christmas...

Mrs. Shively snapped out of this reflective mood, "Now, Doc, you know, next time we see you in March, not February. Carl will have completed four years of therapy. Last year we started a new plan. Every March, you guys would review what was going on with his remission therapy and decide whether Carl should keep taking the 6-mercaptopurine."

No, I didn't know about this March plan and hadn't the foggiest idea what should be done.

There must have been some change in my facial expression, because good old Mrs. Shively looked at me and with a twinkle in her eye said, "Don't worry, Doc, you'll make the right decision."

I watched them leave and reflected on those other moms that Mrs. Shively would call. If anybody would know what to say, at this family time of year, she would.

A radio in the nurses' station was playing Christmas carols.

• • •

I thought the Christmas spirit was dead until Jeff Donaldson was admitted for terminal care that last week of December. Jeff was sitting in a wheelchair, accompanied by the Wagners. Mr. Wagner was pushing the wheelchair, and Jeff was flanked by a girl and boy. When Jeff waved at me, Mrs. Wagner came forward and said, "You must be Jeff's doctor, the one who plays with the soldiers and talks about grandparents." Mrs. Wagner introduced herself and then introduced me to her two children and her husband. After I thanked her for caring for Jeff, she said, "We thought it would be a good experience for our children to share our home with someone at this time of year. But, Doctor, it was good for all of us."

By now, Morgan was in the hall greeting Jeff.

"Are you Morgan or Brigid?" Mr. Wagner asked.

After Morgan introduced herself, Mr. Wagner said, "We know a lot about this place. This must be a very nice children's floor. Jeff is now very weak, and he asked us to bring him back here. If it doesn't interfere, my children would like to spend a little time with him."

"They've each made a small gift for him," Mrs. Wagner said. Tears came to her eyes. "We're going to miss him."

"Of course. There's plenty of time."

The brother said he wanted to push the wheelchair, and the Wagners and Morgan took Jeff to his room.

An hour later, my assessment complete, there was no doubt about terminal care. Jeff's marrow was full of leukemic cells. POMP hadn't prevented a leukemic transformation of his lymphoma. He wasn't eligible for daunomycin, and I decided to do all we could to make him comfortable.

Christmas was on a Friday, so the kids scheduled for monthly POMP that last week of December were admitted a day or two early so they could be discharged on Thursday—home for Christmas Eve.

"Gentle" Jeff Donaldson didn't have a home, at least not in the traditional sense of the word.

• • •

I didn't feel like dashing through National Airport for a flight home to Chicago while the overhead speakers played Christmas carols, and I didn't want to leave Jeff.

I called my parents. After I apologized for not having written or called during the past few weeks, my mother said, "We're pleased you called, Bennett. We know you're busy. You know we'll miss you."

When I explained I was caring for Jeff, my father said, "We read a lot about the troops in Vietnam, but I'm of the opinion you're involved in a different kind of war: one that's more important. We're sorry you can't join us for Christmas. Call anytime. We'd love to know how you're doing."

As I hung up, I thought, how typical of my parents: they weren't pushing me to come home, but they let me know I'd always be welcome.

• • •

In a way, we all were pleased to have Jeff back on 2 East. He was an engaging kid, cooperative and polite. The nurses liked to read to him, and Jeff and I either played with his soldiers or talked of grandparents.

December 24 was a damp, overcast day. I went to a toy store in Rockville to look for a gift for Jeff. I hadn't any idea what he might like. While strolling through the boys' section, I spied a half-size plastic model of an M1 Garand rifle. Jeff's soldiers were of WWII vintage, several holding the M1.

On Christmas Day, Jeff had a number of gifts on his bed, and I added the toy rifle. I initially guessed he liked cookies and small cakes best, but as I visited his room, I began to believe there was something more important going on. On Christmas and the days before, the nurses and even Mrs. Holmquist from social services came to see him—people who liked him and cared for him. For him, being on 2 East was the best part of Christmas morning.

Jeff had found another home, in which he died on December 27.

• • •

I finished my clinical note on Jeff's death. He had died of a rapid progression of sepsis. I closed his chart and sat in the doctors' office.

All the usual cliché about loss went through my mind, but these were quickly displaced by thoughts of what a privilege it had been to know this youngster. He'd been abandoned at birth but then blessed with a loving home for ten years, and he brought joy into the Donaldson home. He'd been welcomed on 2 East and in the Wagner home. He was a gentle soul who in his short stay on 2 East had enriched my life and been "a Child of the Floor" for Brigid, Morgan, Mrs. Holmquist from social services, and the other mothers of 2 East.

I went for a walk. It was winter—gray—and I wasn't dressed for the cold. The turmoil continued. Short phrases came to me: from my childhood, from a few funerals I had attended, from my grandmother's death when my grandfather gave me *Bambi* and my mother read me the entire book. I thought about my exposure as a child to resurrection and eternal life, my readings from Huston Smith and learning of samsara. On and on the random thoughts went. Medical school hadn't been very helpful in this regard. It was one thing to be objective when starting POMP, but now I recognized that emotions were bound to arise during the care of children. It didn't matter whether I tried to remain objective or not.

When I got to the fence, I still wasn't dressed for the weather. My thoughts returned to my parents. "The natural order of things" was OK for grandparents but not for children. They had also counseled me that death was sad, I would miss the deceased, and it was all right to cry.

It was dark. I was cold. I went to bed.

• • •

The next day was devoted to thinking about Jeff. By the twenty-ninth, I was reflecting on how my relationship with Brigid had gone from one of reciprocal professional respect to one of friendship and affection.

After we saw the *Mary Poppins*, Brigid and I continued to date. In October, we decided to see *Behold a Pale Horse*, with Gregory Peck and

Anthony Quinn. It was in black-and-white and a bit grim: not exactly an escape for two people working on 2 East. Over coffee after the film, I said, "I didn't like the dancing. Gregory Peck just can't tap his toes."

Brigid laughed. "Anthony Quinn can't carry a tune, and I can't even recall the title song."

"I'll bet we're the only two people in DC who've gotten a laugh from the film."

Admiring this wonderful human being sitting across the table from me, I asked, "How about next weekend? Have you been to the National Gallery? I haven't. Would you like to go?"

"I'd love to. Yes. I've been there several times. I have to work Saturday; Sunday would be fine."

"Great. It would be nice for me to do something enjoyable for a change rather than mope about Monday morning's admissions, marrows, and POMP."

Brigid nodded but didn't pursue the subject.

• • •

During our stroll through the National Gallery the next Sunday, we often walked hand in hand. While she occasionally took my arm, she rarely called me Ben. Brigid was knowledgeable about the National Gallery, its history, and the collection of paintings, but I had to push for the information; she didn't want to flaunt her interest in art.

"This is how I like to spend my free time: enjoying the benefits of living in a city," Brigid said over dinner. "I gather you like being outdoors in the country."

"Well, you've got that right, but I enjoyed this afternoon. How about going up to Skyline Drive in Shenandoah National Park next weekend?"

"Wonderful. You always insist on paying for dinner, Doctor Humphrey, so I'll pack a picnic lunch next week."

"Weeell, *Nurse* Brigid that would be very nice."

She chuckled. "OK. OK, *Ben.* Shall we start out midmorning?"

"Do you have hiking boots?"

"No, but I have an old pair of white tennis shoes from my student nursing days. We're not going to walk too far, are we?"

When I told her only five miles, we both laughed. We drove back to her apartment: I kissed her good night. "I'm looking forward to our picnic," I said.

She smiled. "Me too."

Our relationship was changing, yet I hadn't found the need to analyze it.

All I knew was that I enjoyed her company, her touch, and her warmth.

• • •

The next Sunday, I picked Brigid up midmorning under a clear sky. "If you'll take this," she said as she handed me a picnic basket, "I'd like to get a scarf and a warm jacket and go over to Virginia with the top down."

With the sun on her face and the wind blowing her scarf, Brigid was a dangerous distraction as we drove over to Shenandoah National Park.

We enjoyed a short hike. On a smooth, flat rock, Brigid opened her basket and displayed a tasty lunch on a red-and-white checkered tablecloth. There were small open-faced sandwiches, a marinated shrimp salad, and, for dessert, a carrot cake.

"I made the cake myself," she said proudly.

We teased one another over lunch until I noticed dark storm clouds to the east moving our way. We drove back to Wisconsin Avenue with the top up. No plans were made for the last weekend in October. Brigid had to work.

When I lifted her chin with a finger to kiss her good night, she put her arms around my neck and stepped in close.

Oh my God—the faint aroma of her perfume and the warmth of her body.

• • •

November and the first two weeks of December were dedicated to coming to terms with Tom Frei's admonishment: I had to accept my responsibilities as a physician. I didn't call Brigid or my parents. I had the company of either Rick or Jerry but not both. I was an asocial creature.

On Wednesday of the third week of December, I asked Brigid if we could go for coffee when she got off work.

"I'd like that."

Before our coffee was served, I stammered, "I'm sorry. I've—I've been a recluse. I should have—I could have called."

She touched my forearm and then took my hand. "It's OK, Ben. I missed not seeing you, but I understand."

Straightening up, infused with some much-needed confidence, I swallowed. She had called me Ben.

Before I could say anything, she continued. "All the nurses are pleased to have all three of you together again."

"It's good to be back."

I didn't know what to say, but Brigid lightened the mood.

"I have a confession to make. I asked Dee if I could help you with Billy Sullivan's marrow, because I wanted to watch you carry him out of the treatment room, and on Tuesday, I eavesdropped on you as Todd talked about Ralph."

After coffee was served, we planned our next rendezvous, agreeing to spend New Year's Eve together at Kirkhill. Frank was going to be visiting his mother.

Spontaneously, words flowed out of my uncensored mind. "You're welcome to spend the night." I corrected my invitation. "No, I'd *like* you to spend the night."

Brigid smiled. "I thought you'd never ask."

• • •

A New Year's Eve date. This year I had one—a very special one, I thought. That was a bit unusual for me. I rarely went out of my way to observe the holiday. Brigid told me she wanted to be responsible for her own prophylaxis and would see a gynecologist. I told her I would also take responsibility for preventing any problems. This wasn't the way Hollywood portrayed such an event. We were two professionals: pregnancy prevention came first; we'd dance in the street, sing a love duet, or find a pink cloud to climb on later.

New Year's Eve at Kirkhill should have started something. We opened a bottle of champagne, sat before a fire, held hands, and snuggled in each other's arms. We talked of previous New Year's Eves, made fun of New Year's resolutions that we had each made in the past, and vowed not to make any that evening. We went to bed at midnight. She was warm and soft, and I enjoyed her touch.

Afterward, we snuggled under the covers, and Brigid said, "I envy you and the other two doctors, Ben. You guys don't have to decide when to quit 2 East. When I started on there, I thought two years would look good on my résumé. I like Washington and want to stay here. Now I'm in my third year; it's like I don't want to abandon the kids. But I think 2 East is wearing me down." She put her head on my shoulder. "And what about you, Doctor Humphrey?"

"In the past, I've always had a five-year plan. Work—lots of work; short breaks in the mountains of the West; and no matrimonial entanglements. I've been selfish and self-centered." Strangely, I now had no plan beyond 2 East, and I didn't care. I knew I needed to finish my training—somewhere in the Midwest or possibly the West.

"Hum." She curled up in my arms.

We fell asleep, two people in a single bed. Two people, each with a problem but not looking for a common path.

Around five, we both woke up.

"How about a cup of coffee, a sweet roll, and a glass of orange juice?"

In predawn light, I drove Brigid to her apartment and kissed her lightly on the mouth. I didn't ask, nor did she inquire about, when we might have another date.

· · ·

I returned to Kirkhill and the fence. Something was wrong. Brigid was likable—more than likable. She had a warm way with people, the kids of 2 East and me. Reflecting on previous end-of-the-year events, I thought this was the most pleasant New Year's—a meaningless holiday— I had ever experienced. But whatever my problem was, sex wasn't the answer—nor was starting a long-term relationship.

I was beginning to feel the emotions of loss. There was Jeff, a "light-foot lad," and Betty Miller, a "rose-lipt maiden." Brigid was also a maiden whom I would never really know.

It was now 1965, the start of a new calendar year. In June, I had said good-bye to my graduate-school years as I left Germany. I didn't know it, but I was now saying good-bye to other things. The idealism of research and the days of short clinical assignments were over. Standing at the fence, I was without a plan. I felt powerless and alone.

JANUARY

First and Second Week

We passed each other in the hall of 2 East and greeted one another. Then Myron turned and called back, "Ben!"

I walked back to him, and he suggested we have a cup of coffee. Myron was my father confessor and fellow traveler down the road of academic life. I always enjoyed his company, so I looked forward to a short break from 2 East.

He asked me how the Christmas holidays had been. I just shrugged.

"I was sorry to learn of the death of Jeff Donaldson," Myron said. "I want to tell you about an impression I have, based on only a few cases. They don't die the week before Christmas; they die the week after Christmas."

"Go on, Myron."

"Well, this is the third kid I've known of who died after Christmas. I can't recall any patient dying just before the holidays. It's as if they find the energy to hang on, enjoy Christmas, and then relax and die." Myron picked up his coffee cup and looked at me. "I wouldn't want to apply statistics to this."

"Well, Myron, I have feelings about the kids of 2 East, about their mothers, about the nurses, about my relationship with Rick and Jerry, and even about Emil J. Freireich that are important to me. They help me get through the day. I never thought of applying statistics to these feelings."

"Good," Myron said. "I thought I'd better add that, you know, just in case you were in an egghead mode."

"Go to hell, Myron." Laughing at myself, I added, "Maybe the egg is no longer hard-boiled."

"I don't think we know if patients can postpone death for a few days, Ben. But what if they can?" Myron shrugged. "What's the biological mechanism for that?"

• • •

"Doctor Humphrey, Tammy's being admitted for bone pain this morning," Brigid said. "They tried to care for her at home, but it just hasn't worked."

Tammy had relapsed the second week in December. She presented with bone pain at that time, and Mrs. Long wanted her treated with daunomycin. It worked. She was pain-free in two days and was discharged before I returned to 2 East on the third week of December. It was still working when I spoke to her by phone the third week of December.

Mrs. Long, another woman, and Tammy, who was sitting, slumped over, in a wheelchair, came down the hall of 2 East at half past eight in the morning.

"Doctor, Tammy's been in such pain at home. It started two weeks ago. We knew it was the leukemia again. Tammy wanted to stay home for Christmas, so our pediatrician tried to keep her pain-free with morphine," Mrs. Long said.

Tears rolled down her cheeks, and she looked spent. I assumed she hadn't slept for several days. "We just want to be here. You'll know how to take care of her, and I'll have the comfort of good nursing," she said, looking at Brigid.

With Brigid's help, I did a very slow and gentle physical exam and then asked, "Can you tell me where it hurts?" I waited. "Can you point to where it hurts?"

No response—only a deep frown. Tammy had winced with every move, so the exam was minimal.

"She hurts all over, Doctor!" a woman standing next to Mrs. Long said in a harsh voice and then louder, "Bone pain! Just like when she was diagnosed, Doctor."

"This is my sister, Jean Selbst," Mrs. Long said. "She's been staying with us to help with Tammy. Jean, this is Doctor Humphrey. He's been very good to Tammy, and this is one of Tammy's favorite nurses, Brigid."

First things first, I thought. Let's see if we can give Tammy relief from her pain and let these two women get some sleep. When I asked about which drugs were given and on what schedule, Mrs. Long gave me a sheet of paper that the visiting nurse had filled out at each home visit.

"That visiting nurse is a real bitch," Miss Selbst said. "That nurse couldn't get in and out of Tammy's bedroom fast enough." Then, louder, "And she gave the morphine when she damn well pleased. And another thing—Tammy's pediatrician doesn't know what he's doing either!"

I asked Brigid to weigh Tammy. She was thirty kilos. From the home-health nurse's sheet, it was obvious that a starting dose of morphine had been ordered, and the schedule varied from four to six hours, a commonly used interval. The starting dose or the lowest recommended dose was too low. Tammy could have received twice as much morphine and at four-hour intervals.

While Brigid and I reviewed Tammy's morphine dose and schedule, Mrs. Long said, "Tammy's pediatrician did care. He came by every day on his lunch hour. He examined—"

"Well, it didn't help with the bone pain, did it!" Miss Selbst interrupted her sister.

"Jean, he did what he could!"

I intervened before Miss Selbst could continue her attack. "Tammy's been getting a dose of morphine on a schedule that is commonly used." I paused, took a deep breath, and continued, "But we can use a different approach. Tammy can receive a higher dose and more frequently."

"Come on, Brigid, let's go talk to the rest of the nursing staff so they all know what's to be done."

Out in the hall, Brigid expressed her disappointment with Tammy's treatment at home. "Tammy's morphine dose was low, and there was no reason to make her wait six hours for the next dose."

"The pediatrician was using a dose of point one milligrams per kilo, and a dose of point two milligrams would still be in the recommended range. However, we can start with a four-hour schedule."

"We sometimes use an every-three-hours interval."

"Thanks. I appreciate knowing that. There's a second priority. Please have social services get a local hotel or motel room with two beds, and let's see if we can get Mrs. Long and the aunt to take turns being with Tammy."

"*The* aunt?" Brigid asked with a smile.

"Mrs. Long is a seasoned veteran of 2 East, and Miss Selbst is just a plebe. What could one expect?" Then I corrected myself and laughed. "OK," I said. "I'm frustrated at Miss Selbst's attitude. There's enough stress even without Tammy's aunt attacking the pediatrician. It doesn't help Mrs. Long to be attacked for defending Tammy's pediatrician."

Brigid drew up the higher dose of morphine and returned to Tammy's room. After writing the admitting orders, I returned to Tammy.

"I gave the morphine at eight fifty," Brigid said.

"Mrs. Long, there should be an effect in twenty minutes."

Miss Selbst looked at her watch.

Oh shit, I thought, I shouldn't have been that precise. So I added, "Sometimes the effect is quicker, and sometimes it takes a little longer."

Tammy was asleep within twenty minutes. To her credit, Miss Selbst convinced her sister that she should rest and insisted on taking the first watch. Forty minutes later, Jean Selbst was snoring in the chair at the bedside.

I went out to feed my buddy Squirrel. What a hell of a way to start the New Year, I thought, as I gave him an extra portion of peanuts.

● ● ●

J erry stopped me in the hall and said he'd heard about Tammy. I suggested we have lunch with Rick.

As we finished our lunch, Rick led the discussion. "During my residency in pediatrics, I got very little training in pain control. Only in my fellowship in hematology/oncology was there any emphasis on treating it."

"Guess that's true in internal medicine, too," Jerry said. "It's the surgeons that taught me about pain." Looking at me, he asked, "Ben?"

I nodded. "Yeah. Well, the cardiologist didn't want any discomfort in a patient with an MI."

"My boss in Minnesota, Krivit, used to say the only pediatricians who knew anything about pain were those taking care of kids with sickle-cell anemia.'"

"Why this lack of interest?" I asked, rather impatiently, remembering the look on Tammy's face.

"Misconceptions?" Rick shrugged. "Kids don't have pain; if they do, they don't remember it. Addiction? Giving narcotics to kids is wrong?"

Disappointment must have been written on my face.

"Probably worst of all, Ben," Rick said, "pain in kids just isn't a priority."

• • •

M organ knocked on the door to the doctors' office. "Hey, Doctor H., Mrs. Long is back from the motel. She looks much better. Tammy's aunt wants to talk to you; I think you'd better see her here in the office. Mrs. Long wants to come along. I'll bring them now, if that's OK.

Five minutes later, Morgan opened the door, and Miss Selbst and Tammy's mother came in. I told Mrs. Long that it looked like some sleep had been good for her. She thanked me and said she was pleased that Tammy had rested while she was gone. I stood up, moved Rick's and Jerry's chair over to my desk, and asked them to sit down.

"How long's she got, Doctor?" Miss Selbst asked. My first thought was, make damn sure you know exactly what she's asking. Miss Selbst repeated herself and then added, "You know, how long is Tammy going to live?"

Well, that answered the question. "I don't know."

"What do you mean you don't know? You're a doctor, aren't you?"

A lot of things flashed through my mind. I remembered Myron saying that kids would hang in there until some important event was over, like a holiday, and then die. I remembered Jeff Donaldson tenaciously hanging on until Christmas was over, or Tommy Paul, who died after he asked his question about how kids get into heaven. Finally, I said, "What I have learned is that kids are tough, but they're also fragile."

"Well, that doesn't answer the question, does it, Doctor," Miss Selbst said. "Maybe I should ask someone with more experience, someone older, someone who isn't afraid to answer the question—"

"Jean!" Mrs. Long frowned and turned toward her sister. She was about to give verbal expression to her anger when I intervened.

"Please, Mrs. Long," I said, waving my hand. "It's OK." I had been told as a medical student that some individuals will take out their frustration on the physician. As an internist, I'd experienced dealing with angry relatives. These individuals are going through hell. If they direct their frustration at you, there's no reason to be defensive; it just comes with the territory.

I turned to Miss Selbst. "I remember a professor of surgery who had decades of experience treating patients with cancer, most of whom died. A medical student asked him when a certain terminal patient was going to die. The surgeon said he didn't know, and when the student persisted in wanting to know, the surgeon simply said, 'I just treat 'em; someone else makes those decisions.'"

"That's good enough for me," Mrs. Long said. "Jean, go get some sleep."

• • •

At Kirkhill that evening, I stood at the fence and wondered about quoting the professor of surgery. I was tired and not formulating things clearly, but I didn't want to think I had used the remark as a cop-out. I had been trained not to forecast a specific time. It wasn't going to be weeks before Tammy would die, but I did feel it was going to be days. How many days, I didn't know, and I was comfortable not knowing.

"Get some sleep," Mrs. Long had said. I took her advice and went to bed.

• • •

Friday afternoon before I left for Kirkhill, I went to see Tammy. Mrs. Long and Morgan were applying makeup. All three were enjoying this undertaking. Tammy's face was pied: red cheeks, a blue hue under the eyes, and brown eyebrows, all in contrast to the pallor of anemia. They stopped, but I asked them to please continue. When a mirror was held up, a smile came over her face. She used what little energy she had to nod.

"I was so disorganized this week when we came into the hospital that I didn't think to bring her makeup kit," Mrs. Long said. "But Jean and I put a few things together this morning."

Morgan stepped aside so I could come closer to Tammy. "Great idea." I was taken by the way Tammy looked at me, as if she were saying thanks.

As I stood in the rain that night at the fence, I didn't formulate anything specific. That was now happening much of the time.

After I called 2 East to check on Tammy early Saturday morning, I poked around the cabin in the predawn darkness, brewed coffee, and baked some cinnamon rolls. While waiting for daybreak, I opened my Untermeyer anthology and looked for something to read. Generally, I read poetry late at night. I remembered using *pied* in thinking about Tammy's face, a word I had learned from Hopkins's poem "Pied Beauty." So I read the section on Gerard Manley Hopkins. The poems were peaceful but not especially relevant to Tammy's condition. The text contained an interesting passage: "He delighted in 'couple-colored' oddities." An interesting parallel, I thought: artificial color on a terminal face.

At 8:10 a.m., I was back on 2 East and checked with the nurses; Tammy was comatose. She was my only kid in the hospital. I hung around 2 East, cleaning my desk, filing reprints. At 10:25 a.m. Tammy was gone. Morgan and Mrs. Long were at her bedside when she died. Now the bright colors of makeup lay on an ashen face.

● ● ●

Rick came into the office as I was writing the final note in Tammy's chart. I nodded when he asked if Tammy had died.

"I liked her. And her mom, too. I got to know her when you were off the floor those first two weeks in December. The makeup—what a neat distraction," Rick said.

"That's what I thought too. But Morgan gave me a different slant on that. She reminded me that Tammy desperately wanted to be a teenager. Morgan feels that because Tammy got to wear perfume, makeup, and a pretty nightgown and we all looked at her fashion magazines this ten-year-old preadolescent got to be a teenager, got to be what she wanted to before she died."

Rick sat back in his chair and put his fingers together. "I think Morgan got that right."

Third and Fourth Week

Monday morning, Billy "Bear" Sullivan and Dan Martin were both admitted and in their rooms by nine. I hadn't given Dan a nickname yet. During his December admission, I had noted that Dan would pat his mother's arm as she wrestled with the diagnosis. When I walked in, Morgan was taking his temperature. After I said good morning, Mrs.

Martin volunteered, "Dan's back to being himself again. I even wondered if we needed to come in this morning."

Morgan and I looked at each other. "That's typical of kids in remission from leukemia."

Fifteen minutes later I carried a weeping Dan back to his mother and explained, "I'll be back after I look at Dan's marrow."

When Mrs. Martin told me she hoped it would be normal, I said, "I hope it'll be a *remission* marrow, not containing any readily identifiable leukemia cells. There's a difference between a marrow in remission from leukemia and a normal marrow. Mrs. Martin, we can talk about that later this morning."

"But if he doesn't have leukemia, we don't have to talk about it, do we?"

"I'm sorry, Mrs. Martin. Other mothers have told me how difficult these first weeks are. There are a lot of complicated things about diagnosing and treating leukemia. It's my responsibility to explain all this to you."

As I walked out, I felt weak. This poor mother. I needed to talk to someone. Mrs. Sullivan! First things first, Humphrey. Let's make sure Billy's in remission, and then maybe Mrs. Sullivan can share some of her experience in trying to help Dan's mother.

"No bad cells." I told Mrs. Sullivan the good news forty-five minutes later. After she gave Billy a hug, I said, "I appreciate your talking to Mrs. Martin last month."

"Oh, Doctor Humphrey, I can't communicate with Virginia Martin. I tried last month while we were here on the floor together, and I called her once at home. I just made her nervous: one denial after another."

I thanked her for trying.

"I remember that first week: the anger, the irrational thoughts. I wanted to wrap Billy in a blanket and go hide." Tears streamed down her cheeks.

This was my pragmatic mom, my "Oh, you just adapt" mother. You need to remember this, Humphrey. Most will adapt, but you must be patient during that first week while they are trying to adjust to the hell of this diagnosis.

I apologized for having asked her to help and said I was sorry for the pain that had been reawakened.

"Oh no. I got through it all due to support from other mothers. Anytime, anytime. Just ask me, and I'll gladly help," she said.

I walked slowly down to Dan's room. Dan and his mother were playing with a xylophone. Mrs. Martin put it on the bed, picked up her son, and put him on her lap. She smiled when I told her about the remission state. "Well, maybe he didn't have leukemia after all."

I tried to explain.

"Couldn't we *not* give him the drugs to see if he really does have leukemia?"

With each statement of denial and my attempted explanation, Mrs. Martin twisted her hands, and a noticeable tremor rose in her voice. Initially, Dan was indifferent to the discussion, squirming as kids do. Now he was looking at his mom and patted her arm. I decided to dub him Dan "Supportive" Martin.

Dan and I played with the xylophone for a few minutes, and as I left his room, I thought, what the hell are you going to do next, Doctor?

• • •

I entered Dee's office. She took one look at me and said, "It's about Mrs. Martin, isn't it?"

I asked if she was clairvoyant. Dee explained, "Morgan's also worried."

"Well, Morgan's right on." After a brief review of my verbal interactions and observations of the morning with Mrs. Martin, I asked Dee if this kind of denial was common.

"Sometimes during the first remission, but after five days of POMP and a chance for the mother of the newly diagnosed child to meet and talk to other mothers, there's acceptance. In my experience, Mrs. Martin is unusual."

When I explained that Mrs. Sullivan hadn't been able to help, Dee noted that Mrs. Martin didn't join the other mothers during rest hour.

"I'll talk to her and ask Barbara to chat with her. Maybe a few gray hairs will help. I'll let you know if we make any progress."

"Thanks, Dee. I feel better. But then, you are after all our Mother Superior."

• • •

Sign-out rounds for the three clinical associates of 2 East were easy. None of the kids would receive POMP over the weekend.

"Think of all the time we're saving not spending Monday deciding who will get a chest x-ray on Tuesday," I quipped. I glanced warily at both clinical associates. We'd all had to sit out our two weeks, and it hadn't been easy for any of us.

Jerry raised an eyebrow. "Yeah," he said. "No soul-searching for whether this kid or that kid is a greater risk."

Rick shook his head. "So much for my training from Minnesota," he said. Jerry and I exchanged a glance. Therapy delay had been an irrational response to emotional stress. Rick would keep his kids on schedule, but the past was still on his mind. "I just hope we get through the next six months without another Jennifer Johnson," he said.

"Can we really be sure POMP was solely to blame for that?" I asked. "OK. It had something to do with methotrexate, sure. But did Jennifer's makeup include a minor abnormality in folic-acid metabolism, maybe? Or was it just odds that this type of toxicity would occur in one in one hundred thousand kids with leukemia? Who knows?"

"One in a million is one too many, Ben," Rick said.

Jerry interrupted us. "OK, you two. I don't know if one can spend too much time doing clinical pediatrics and get too involved with kids, but, Ben, I think you've spent too much time in the lab."

I chuckled. "I'll accept that. But I too don't ever want to see another Jennifer. No matter what the explanation."

Everybody nodded. Even I could feel the internal turmoil around drug toxicity that still resided in me. Rick had stated it openly, but I felt that Jerry and I were not expressing our feelings. For the last three months, POMP had been given on schedule, and that was the way it was going to be.

• • •

All year there was a steady influx of new patients, and January was no exception. Rick and Jerry had both recently admitted newly diagnosed cases, so I wasn't surprised to see an unfamiliar name on the Board for me Monday afternoon.

"Your new admission is here, Doctor H.," Morgan said. "Joshua Anderson is ten and armed. Be careful." She smiled.

As I entered Joshua's room, I found myself looking down the barrel of a full-size toy model Colt 45, held by a thin redheaded boy. I put my hands up, and he smiled. His mother stood, closed her Bible after carefully marking her place, looked patiently at her son, and gently took the revolver. There must have been four other guns on the bed plus five or six comic books, all Westerns.

"You must be Doctor Humphrey," Mrs. Anderson said. She was in her early thirties and wore a full-length dress and an open cardigan, which revealed a golden cross. "Our doctor give me this," she said, handing me a business-size envelope that bore a red logo: "Saint Andrew's Memorial Hospital."

There was a description of Joshua's medical history of anemia, physical findings of an enlarged spleen, and a pathology report describing the morphology of the peripheral blood, immature lymphocytes, decreased platelets, and reduction in the number of red blood cells.

"This is an excellent summary and very helpful," I said. Before I started to take a history or explain our procedures, I thought I'd better pay some attention to Joshua. I asked him to "give me five" and got a good slap in return. Joshua's gaze was steady, and his whole deportment suggested he'd be good in any scrap with a kid his own age.

"My dad's a sheriff," Joshua said proudly. His mother corrected him, saying he was a deputy sheriff. "Yes, ma'am," Joshua said.

When I asked if he preferred "Josh," his mother informed me that it was "Joshua." I was struck that both mom and son addressed me as "sir" and any yes-or-no response made by Joshua to his mother always ended in "ma'am."

Mrs. Anderson was laconic, plainspoken, and pleasant—a no-nonsense type of person. When I returned with the results of the aspiration and explained our policy of telling the kids the name of their disease, Mrs. Anderson said, "We don't lie to Joshua, and he don't lie to us."

I decided to play it straight with these two, take my time to get to know how to best communicate, and not attempt humor. It was January, and I wasn't in a humorous mood anyway.

• • •

Morgan had forewarned me that Mrs. Graham had called this morning. "John had been sick to his stomach for a few days and now has petechiae. John's father was going to take the week off from work to help. They'll be here this afternoon."

"Sick to his stomach"—that could mean a return of his abdominal tumor. Petechiae could mean leukemic conversion of his lymphoma. By the time you get all that straightened out, it might be after five in the evening. Organize the treatment options this morning so I don't have to tell the Grahams that they have to wait until tomorrow to discuss therapy.

First, I called radiation therapy.

"We'll pull John Graham's chart. You can come down right away," a receptionist said.

The waiting area of the radiation- therapy department was gruesome. By definition, all the patients receiving radiotherapy had some sort of cancer. An elderly man sitting in a wheelchair had a nasogastric tube hanging from his nose; black marks on his neck indicated the radiation field. He hadn't shaved for weeks, and I assumed he had a carcinoma in the neck. A woman in her forties was also in a wheelchair. The institutional bathrobe didn't conceal a swollen left arm, a case of lymph edema caused by node dissection for breast cancer. Finally there was a man on a gurney, bald with black marks on his skull—a brain tumor, I presumed. "God," I thought, "did John see patients like these while getting radiation back in July? No wonder he's terrified."

The receptionist led me back to a conference room. Hanging from a view box was an x-ray of an abdomen. A middle-aged man introduced himself. He had reviewed John's course of radiotherapy, and if we wished, he could receive additional radiation to the abdomen. He went on to say that as this was probably a case of leukemic conversion, John would require chemotherapy, but radiotherapy could again be used to relieve any obstruction.

I called Freireich's office and told his secretary I had a problem with one of my kids that I wanted to discuss. I was told to come right up. I'll give Jay credit, I thought. If we needed to see him, he was always available.

"What do you want to do?" Jay asked after I told him about what I knew about John.

I outlined a number of options. My main question was whether Jay wanted him on the daunomycin protocol.

"No. That protocol is limited to patients with ALL and not lymphomas with leukemic conversation."

"If the parents did want to continue treatment, we could try cyclophosphamide, but I'd like to know if you had a better idea," I said.

"Cyclophosphamide's a good choice."

"I'm sorry to trouble you with this discussion when I don't have more data," I said. "I just didn't want to be in the position at five o'clock of finding out it's a relapse and then having to tell the mother that we'd discuss treatment the next day after rounds." Then I added, "He's kind of a sad kid and has a very good mom."

"No," Jay said slowly, "I understand; you just want to do the best you can for this family. Besides, five o'clock is never a problem. You can always call me at home."

I thanked him and left. As I walked down the hall, I thought, the whole scene in Jay's office had been weird. I was prepared for him to be apathetic. Instead he was sympathetic to me and my problem.

• • •

The Grahams walked onto 2 East at 3:20 p.m. Mr. Graham was tall and built like a football player. He was carrying John in his arms.

"This is Doctor Humphrey," Mrs. Graham said.

"I appreciate the interest you've shown in my son," Mr. Graham said.

I didn't quite know how to respond. "You're welcome" didn't seem appropriate, so I commented that I knew that he had been helpful to John and his mother.

"We've all worked hard," Mr. Graham said.

John had petechiae on his trunk and extremities, a soft abdomen, and a palpable spleen two inches below the left costal margin. There were normal bowel sounds, and I could not feel an abdominal mass.

Thank God, I thought, no need for radiation therapy. John had an elevated temperature, so in addition to blood counts and chemistries, I drew a blood culture. I took a very brief history and told the Grahams I wanted to look at John's blood and be back as soon as possible.

Up in the path lab, I didn't have to look for leukemic cells: they were all over the place. It was hard to find any normal white cells or platelets.

Both parents just nodded when I told them; they already knew. During the interim history, I was impressed that Mr. Graham understood a great deal about platelets, marrow suppression, and relapse. "Mr. Graham, you seem to understand all of this technical stuff."

"Julia has explained all this. She's very knowledgeable."

"That's because Doctor Humphrey and all the nurses have spent time with me. And Mary Sue Thompkins, Kathryn Sullivan, and I have become good friends. Mary Sue taught me about the drugs, and Billy was here getting platelets that first week when John was receiving radiation therapy." She paused. "I know about you and Billy's teddy bear."

To bring Mr. Graham into the conversation, I said, "I know about the stock-car races, the visit by John's grandfather, and you trying to help your son fall asleep."

"I've taken this week off from work. I'll do whatever I can. After all, he's my only son." He looked at his wife and added, "*Our* only son."

Mrs. Graham reached over and took his hand.

I went over the treatment options. They had already decided that they just wanted John to be comfortable.

"I just hope it will be pain-free," Mrs. Graham said.

• • •

The next day, I was in the hall, looking at the Board, when Mrs. Graham asked, "May I see you for a minute?" She was on her way out for a much-needed break.

We went down to the doctors' office.

She said she appreciated the time I spent yesterday talking to John's father.

"Well," I said, "I had to tell him I wasn't a dad but that I could remember being a young son. I liked hearing about the stock-car races, the three Graham men sitting together. That reminded me of sitting in the rain fishing with my father and grandfather. It was on the Pere Marquette Lake near Ludington, Michigan—a chance to know my place in a lineage."

"Helen Miller asked me to say hello to the nurses and Doctor Sandler," Mrs. Graham said.

I asked how Mrs. Miller was doing.

"We'll, she has her ups and downs," Mrs. Graham said. "But she also has a small group of mothers from 2 East who call her or whom she can call. Boy, I sure appreciate talking to her." Then she added, "I hope Jennifer Johnson's mom…"

For one mom to talk to another who's been through a death was a kind of help beyond my imagination. But these maternal support systems didn't have to be about bad things. "Lucky" Carl was a long-term survivor, yet his mother still had a support circle of 2 East friends.

I noted tears on Mrs. Graham's cheeks. It was the first time I had seen her cry.

"I feel sorry for John's father," she said. "He doesn't have anyone else to talk to."

• • •

John Graham died at 11:37 p.m.

• • •

January had been a dismal and dreary month, but it wasn't over yet. Dee met me in the hall. I was struck by the urgency of her message. "Doctor Humphrey, there's a call for you. Mr. Yardley."

"Mr. Yardley?"

She nodded. Odd, I thought, and hoped that nothing had happened to Todd's mom.

"Doctor Humphrey, this is Tom Yardley, Todd's father." In an emotionally choked voice, Mr. Yardley continued. "Todd died this afternoon; he fell down the stairs. We heard the fall and one scream. When we got to him, he was unconscious. He started to have fits in the car. They did a spinal in the ER. There was blood in the fluid. Then he died." A long pause. "He never woke up."

I don't remember what I said. I do remember Mr. Yardley mentioning Todd's stories of 2 East, something about his appreciation of all we had done for Todd. I said how fond I was of his son. "The nurses all liked Todd," I said. I ascertained the time of the fall, the name of the hospital, and the time of death.

I sat at my desk, looking at the facts I needed to write into Todd's medical record.

The phone rang again. "Doctor Humphrey, Tom Yardley. I forgot to tell you we agreed to an autopsy. We know that you're doing research, and if we could learn something…" Then he added, "Well, that might help some child in the future."

January, 28, 1965

Mr. Yardley called to report the death of his son, Todd.

Todd Yardley (b. March 9, 1958) was diagnosed on April 14, 1964. He achieved a remission after one course of POMP and has received monthly courses through December 1964.

Presumptive cause of death: Trauma to head with resulting cerebral hemorrhage. The patient fell down a flight of stairs at 2:15 p.m., unconscious immediately thereafter; seizures observed approximately 2:30 p.m.; a lumbar puncture performed at Saint Joseph's Hospital ER revealed hemorrhagic spinal fluid. Patient died at 2:45 p.m. This accident occurred at the nadir of thrombocytopenia after a course of POMP.

Parents agreed to postmortem exam.

G. Bennett Humphrey, MD Clinical Associate, 2 East

When I signed my note, I thought about how little it told of an endearing six-year-old boy, his relationship with his mother, and his friend Ralph.

• • •

January. Tammy Long had died; daunomycin had stopped her bone pain, so she could be home for Christmas. John Graham died after months of POMP, an antileukemic therapy that wasn't designed for lymphomas.

My kids scheduled for monthly therapy came in on Monday. They were all in remission, and I wrote the POMP orders in the late morning; that was my job. The nurses hung the bags of drugs for infusion; that was their task. Jay Freireich would collect the charts and determine if the toxicity induced by POMP was acceptable; that was his responsibility. My time away from the kids had helped me see that, even though our actions were well-meaning, there was no excuse for altering the protocol. By delaying POMP therapy, we were trying to give kids the chance to resist the toxicity of the drugs. But what if our delays had caused kids to relapse? It wasn't our choice to make. And by changing the protocol, we had risked the integrity of the research.

I was beginning to understand that the enemy of 2 East was not POMP but leukemia. If we were ever going to cure this disease, there was a lot of work to be done. Yes, children would die. Some of them, like Jennifer Johnson, would die from the horrible toxicity of POMP. But without carefully, methodically establishing the efficacy of the drug therapy, there was to no way to beat leukemia.

FEBRUARY

First and Second Week

I drove to work in the awakening dawn, but I always returned to Kirkhill in the dark. Mondays were always darker than every other day. The shortest month of the year was short of sunlight, and spring seemed a long way off.

The kids brightened my day, and I would come out of my shell listening to Sally "Doctor Humpfee" Carter, or asking Billy Sullivan about Bear, or being charmed by one of Robert "Gosh" Thurman's tales of his new puppy, or accepting Sarah Thompkins's polite hostility. But in between listening, putting puzzles together, and reading a book aloud, time turtled along; some days seemed never to end.

On rare occasions, I would pass a certain door on 2 East and remember, that's the room where Tommy Paul asked, "How do kids get into heaven?" Or the place where Jeff Donaldson accepted a spoonful of spinach from Morgan. Where Tammy last wore makeup. Generally, the hall was just long and poorly lit, and each door had only a number.

• • •

Feeding the animals daily was a break from this dismal pace. I liked being told to hurry up by an impatient equine or hear the quiet yelp of "Let me out" or a bark of "Let me in" by Shonto.

One day in early February, I went out in a drizzle with a bag of peanuts and turned around before I reached my bench. On the wet pavement was a tuft of matted red fur, a twisted flattened body with a long bushy tail.

I went for a long walk. This was a death I had to deal with right now; I didn't feel like I could put it off, wait for time at the fence. An unexpected death. Was it any different from the expected deaths of 2 East? The death of kids hurt, and so did this loss of my buddy Squirrel. It just didn't seem fair.

Death of patients goes with your profession, Humphrey. Death of a friend goes with life.

• • •

The flow of aerograms slowed. That was my fault. In November, I wrote Kristina that I didn't see how I could possibly go skiing in Germany this year. It was the only time I commented on my clinical responsibilities. They were not part of my relationship with Kristina. When we were dating, I was working in a laboratory. I arrived on time in the morning and left at five. I never brought problems from the lab to my evenings or my weekends. To Kristina, I was a free spirit.

I wrote her about the beauty of the rolling hills of Maryland, the tranquility of Kirkhill, the training of a Thoroughbred, and the enfolding of summer's green followed by the colors of fall. They were emotionally important to me, a third of my time, and easy to share. Kristina and I shared the forest above the Rhine and the Bavarian Alps. We had these and other places in common.

I could have written about my comradeship with Rick and Jerry, how important they were to me. She had introduced me to her fellow graduate students, and we spent evenings together sharing a bottle of wine. There seemed to me to be a difference. Her social interactions with these acquaintances were verbal. My time with Rick and Gerry was mostly nonverbal, and I called them my friends.

I never wrote about the children of 2 East, the last third of my time but 80 percent of my emotional life. My skills weren't up to describing the pleasure of holding Michele Karr on my lap, the compassion of carrying a sobbing Billy Sullivan out of the treatment room, or the privilege of knowing Jeff Donaldson. This was a private world and 2 East an ineffable place.

On a rainy Sunday night in mid-January, I wrote a series of phrases and questions on scrap paper. Next year I'd be in the lab, but after that there would be one year of residency and then two years of fellowship. I wrote down, "Humphrey, you know how hard you can work, how you are willing to keep long hours and work on weekends to ensure success." What kind of life would that be for her? Kris is getting a PhD, preparing for a career. You're a workaholic. Kris enjoyed your company when you were a free spirit. I looked at that scrap of paper. It was as if I were choosing to end my relationship with Kristina, not to subject her to being neglected in a foreign land. If all the stuff on the scrap of paper was bullshit, what was the truth? I really didn't know. I lacked the emotional energy to pursue any relationship outside of my commitments on 2 East. Or maybe thinking of a future with an attractive wife of German origin, living together while I pursued a career in academic medicine, just didn't fit with who I was, or at least who I was at present.

I vividly recall throwing the scrap of paper away. The rain and wind continued. I wrote Kristina telling her that, upon finishing her graduate work, I hoped she would get the faculty position she wanted. It was a "Dear Jane" letter, but I really did wish the best for her.

In mid-February, on a dark Wednesday night, the last aerogram from Kristina lay upon the table, her "Dear John" letter to me. She reminded me of special evenings, especially a costume party during carnival when I came dressed as Faust and she as a Bavarian princess. She wrote about our ski trip and our favorite *weinstube* in Bingen where we liked to go after hiking on the opposite shore of the Rhine. She too wished me well and thanked me for being her friend.

My year in Germany had been very full, and the brightest light was Kristina. I stored this aerogram with previous letters and photos of our time together.

My lonely mood accompanied me to the fence. As usual, I searched for a poem or a folk song to fit my feelings. I remembered the musical *Bells Are Ringing* starring Judy Holliday. Near the end of the film, wearing a red dress and alone on stage, she sang "The Party's Over." I could almost hear Judy's voice. I could paraphrase the words as if they were a poem, and I spoke them to Domino: "The party's over. / The candles flicker and dim. / You danced and dreamed through that year, / it seemed to be right just being with her. / Now you must wake up, all dreams must end. / Take off your makeup. The party's over. / It's all over, my friend."

• • •

On Thursday, the second week of February, Dee told me there was a new admission, a ten-year-old named Polly Sorensen. I hadn't had a new kid to treat for several weeks, and my caseload was a little low due to several deaths, so I thought of this new admission as a sort of re-placement kid. As I walked to the room, I wondered, a replacement for whom? Jeff Donaldson? Todd Yardley? Tammy Long?

Polly walked over to greet me. "Hi, I'm Polly. These are for you," she said, handing me several sheets of her medical records. That was unusu-al; where was the anxiety, the fear or uneasiness about being in a strange place? Polly was not thin—more wiry or lean. Her dark-red hair lay in dis-array, and she had attractive bright eyes. She wore bib overalls, a T-shirt, and gym shoes. There was something handsome about this outgoing kid. She sized me up and concluded, "You must be Doctor Humphrey."

"Come over here, Polly," Mrs. Sorensen said, in a manner suggesting she was used to dealing with her outgoing daughter. They were a pair of opposites; Mom had a soft, pretty appearance, with long blond hair and wore a gray dress.

"I've been worried about Polly for the last week or two. She is never willing to admit she's sick. She doesn't want anything to interfere with visiting her friends – even she has a winter cold," Mrs. Sorensen said in a quiet, slow, manner. "I prefer..."

"Yes, mom, but we worked that out," Polly inserted. She turned, looked at me, and explained, "During the winter months, I let mom take my temperature any time she's worried. If, I have a fever, I stay home, but I get to call my friends and talk on the phone as long as I want to. It's not nice to pass germs onto good friends."

Charming, extroverted, and spontaneous, I could imagine that this ten-year-old tomboy was a hand-full at home.

"For the last week or so, Polly hasn't been very active, her appetite is down and I've notice some increase in the size of her stomach. She didn't want to take time out from her activities to go see a doctor, but this morning I noticed little red dots on her arms.

Polly popped off the bed and showed me her arms. "It's just a rash, Doctor Humphrey."

Mrs. Sorensen then related: the emergency appointment with their doctor, finding of an enlarged spleen, the laboratory test that revealed leukemia in Polly's blood, and that Polly was told an admission to NIH rather than the local hospital was necessary.

"I want to go to the playroom and meet some of the other kids," Polly said to her mother.

"Ask Doctor Humphrey, Polly."

"I want to go to the playroom and meet some . . ."

"Polly" her mother said in a tone that Polly apparently understood.

There was a pause and a reformulation. "Doctor Humphrey, *may* I go to the playroom and meet some of the other kids?" she asked in a more formal manner.

I suggested, we get the bone marrow aspiration out of the way, establish the diagnosis, let me look at some laboratory tests, and then I would personally introduce her to Robert Thurman. "He is a bit younger than you, but he is very knowledgeable about leukemia. You two can talk, and he'll take you around and introduce you to some of the other kids who also have leukemia.

As if the lights had just been turned on, Polly brightened up with a smile. I assumed, she had considered NIH as an interruption in her life. Now, it was a social opportunity, new friends to make, unique friends - kids like her that also had leukemia.

So I met Polly—not a replacement kid but a vibrant individual.

Third and Fourth Week

On the Board, under my name, was Dan Martin, four years old. It should have been Dan "Supportive" Martin, but the nurses didn't know the nicknames of my patients.

As I walked into Dan's room, I wondered how Mrs. Martin was dealing with the diagnosis of leukemia. Dan was sitting next to his mother, and the two were looking at a Mickey Mouse book. She looked up as I greeted Dan, and by the time I said good morning, she had closed the book. She sat up straight and put her hands together, one grasping the other. Bad body language, I thought. I sat down in the extra metal chair.

When I asked Dan if he'd show me his book, he came over with a smile and opened it. We boys looked at Mickey, Donald, and Pluto. He liked Goofy best. After a few minutes, I noticed Mrs. Martin sat back in the armchair and unclasped her hands.

"Dan, you know all these animals. That's very good," I said.

"He loves books," Mrs. Martin said. "We've read this Mickey Mouse multiple times."

I asked, "How's Dan been at home since the last treatment?" Again she sat up straight and clasped her hands. Dan went over to his mother.

When I returned later in the morning with the good news about a remission marrow, Dan again stood by his mom. As I walked out of his room, I remembered he was "Supportive" Dan.

Dan and I spent the rest of the week looking at and talking about books or playing with the xylophone. As long as I didn't push the language of leukemia with Mrs. Martin, she was at ease. I understood that was the best way for me to be supportive, something I'd learned from Dan.

When it came to caring for Dan, that was the way the rest of my year went—March, April, May, and June. On the third Monday, I never asked about signs or symptoms of leukemia; I just did the bone-marrow aspirate and informed Mrs. Martin it was "good." It was the only thing I could do.

• • •

Wednesday night at the fence, I pondered Dan. Dee hadn't made any progress in talking to Mrs. Martin. Was there anything wrong with Mrs. Martin's coping style? All of us assumed this denial caused Dan's mother extra stress; maybe we were right, but maybe it was what Mrs. Martin had to do. I didn't know. Dee told me she didn't think it was healthy, but in fact she didn't know.

• • •

On Thursday, I talked to Myron about Dan's mom.

"I think you're right; we *don't* know. We talk about coping styles: information avoiders and information seekers. With Mrs. Martin, you're dealing with denial versus acceptance." His comments were typical of his philosophical style and why I liked to discuss problems with him. "It's reassuring to a physician to think he knows what he's doing. That assumption closes the door on learning anything," Myron said. "But in this arena of psychological support, informed consent, and coping styles, if you say you don't know, then you can work with a psychologist and try to find out."

• • •

On a Sunday evening, the phone rang at Kirkhill. "Hi, Ben, this is Paula," a familiar voice said.

"Paula!" I said in a crescendo of rising delight.

We exchanged the usual questions and answers. To my surprise, Paula was still not married, so when she asked if I'd like to come up to Philadelphia for a weekend, I said yes. During the upcoming week, I could clear my calendar and make sure I had coverage for the hospital. Frank could take care of the horses.

When I hung up the phone, memories revived. I met Paula on a March ski trip sponsored by the University of Chicago on my last spring break before my postdoc in Germany. She was a brunette with a slender athletic figure, playful and capricious but too tall to be a pixie. I couldn't outski her and didn't want to. Occasionally I fell on some difficult runs, but Paula never did. She teased me about who was the better skier. After skiing together for a few days, I asked if I could take her picture. I helped her assume a pose and then pushed her down into the snow and took her picture, saying I'd label it "Paula trying to ski an intermediate run." After she mocked a protest, I helped her up only to be pushed into a snowbank, have my picture taken, and be told, "I'll label this 'Ben on a bunny run.'"

I was enchanted. It turned out she was also intelligent and interested in music and art.

Paula was a senior, majoring in art history, graduating in June. We would graduate together, she receiving a BA and I my PhD, but in March that was in the distant future. More ominous was that, after a postdoctoral year in Germany, I would be a commissioned officer in the US Public Health Service for two years. Paula's charm made these commitments irrelevant. It was a hiatus from my tightly controlled workaholic schedule, and I was in love.

Standing at the fence, I recalled that spring in 1963: intense, passionate dating, strolls through local art fairs, and afternoons sailing on Lake Michigan.

There was one evening, especially memorable, when my information-hungry mind destroyed an artistic moment. "I've learned to play a soprano recorder," Paula said.

"How about a concert?"

"OK, but the recorder is a delicate instrument. Promise me you won't bring your trumpet."

"Deal."

Two days later, in a cloister attached to one of the ivy-covered gothic buildings, I was told where to stand, and Paula took her special place. While the music flowed, I focused on the structure, the scales, and the clarity of the instrument. The sound was pleasant, but not knowing anything about the recorder, I asked, "What's the range of the instrument?"

Paula exploded in a forte of rage. I still remember what she said: "I've practiced this piece in hallways, entranceways, and alcoves all over this campus. This cloister is perfect for resonance. It brings out the overtones and enriches the sound, and you, *you* want to know the range of the instrument!"

I remember taking her in my arms and telling her I was sorry. I thought then and especially this evening two years later, how could I have been such a klutz?

Like all my graduate-school friends, Paula was a frequent guest in my parents' home, but a very special one as far as my mother was concerned.

After her first Sunday visit, my mother said, "Now, Bennett, you make sure to bring Paula back next Sunday. I'm fixing a ham with a pineapple sauce."

"I'd like that. Thank you," Paula said.

It was something I was glad to do, but that didn't matter. I was standing between two very important women.

Later my mother told me, "Oh, Bennett, I could just take that little Paula to my heart." Paula was taller than mom, and the *little* was a term of endearment.

When John, a friend who had been on the March ski trip, found out I was going to Germany and that Paula wasn't going along, he told me, "Marry that girl or cancel your goddamn trip to Europe and spend next year courting that girl or I'll beat the shit out of you."

John was a lot bigger than me, more colorful in his speech, and very astute.

Now, in February 1965, I was trying to focus on an opportunity to see a very special person. This was a moment to get away from the dull 2 East hallway and the bright surgical lights of the soundproof room at the end of the hall.

It was overcast: no stars and no moon. It was difficult to see.

• • •

The only easy part of the week was making the plans. Frank would care for the horses, and Jerry would cover the weekend.

"It's about time you got out of here," Jerry said. "You didn't take any time off at Thanksgiving or Christmas, and you canceled your ski trip to Europe." When I pointed out that Rick hadn't taken any time off either, Jerry looked at me with a solemn expression and said, "Yeah—but he's saving up time for when the baby's born. You don't have an excuse."

Why hadn't I taken time off? Vacations into the outdoors were a hallmark of my graduate-school days. I was smart enough to know I needed to get away for a week or two, and I enjoyed being away from the long hours and extreme effort. To break loose was part of my plan in those days. Now, I didn't have a plan. I was bound to this place, this floor full of kids where the hours weren't long but the effort was intense. Well, I thought, I can ski next year.

The gloom of Monday morning's bone marrows passed, as all our kids were in remission. Penny "the Biter" Tapley, my defiant two-year-old, arrived in the afternoon. Looking at her marrow, I felt gloom give way to despair. There weren't any leukemic cells; there just weren't many normal cells. The marrow hadn't recovered from the previous course of POMP. In the peripheral blood count, no granulocytes. I showed the results to Rick, who shook his head slowly and said that he, too, was giving POMP on Monday to kids with low counts. Jerry asked me if Penny had had any problems with sepsis in the past, and I said no.

• • •

Penny was alone. She neither wanted nor accepted the emotional care the nurses offered. If Penny was lonesome or felt abandoned, I never recognized it. She put her energy into defiantly defending her private space. Most of the time, the mood in Penny's room felt drab. On admission, Morgan had brought a few brightly colored stuffed animals from the playroom and placed them on Penny's bed. She ignored the animals and Morgan. Because she would pull out her IV given a chance, her arms and legs were wrapped in gauze and pinned to the bed. It was as if she were lying on an immovable rack.

Tuesday morning on rounds, I found Brigid wiping Penny's mouth and talking to her. Asking Brigid to help me with the exam, I went over every inch of Penny's skin as well as performed the usual palpation of the abdomen and auscultation of the chest. Then, we pinned Penny back to the bed.

As we walked together toward the nurses' station, Brigid said, "We try to spend as much time with her as possible." I told her I appreciated that, even if Penny didn't. "We try to prolong mealtime; Penny really likes to eat. We know she's overweight; she gets lots of snacks, especially puddings. I hope you don't mind."

"No, of course not. Does the chemotherapy interfere with her joy of eating?" I was told that the staff didn't offer Penny food with the infusion of some drugs but that most of the time Penny readily ate. "A spoonful of food can go a long, long way."

Brigid went into the nurses' station; I went down to the doctors' office. Down the hall in her room, Penny stared at the ceiling.

• • •

While Tuesday was uneventful, my fear was realized when Penny spiked a fever Wednesday afternoon. Blood cultures were drawn and antibiotics started, which meant Penny was going to be in the hospital for the weekend. Now my anxiety included the reality that Penny might die in a day or two, or within a week. I could have been optimistic and assumed it was just a virus, but there were virtually no white cells in Penny's peripheral blood.

To complicate matters, I was in the doldrums the whole week. If I had had the insight, I would have known that I'd been in a slump since November. To make matters worse, I was now in a quandary about Philadelphia. I wasn't sure I could leave 2 East and enjoy myself. I didn't think I'd be very good company. Would I be in Philadelphia with a twenty-three-year-old woman but overtly preoccupied with a two-year-old in Bethesda?

Jerry was an excellent physician and could provide as good care as any physician—maybe better. Furthermore, neither I nor the nursing staff had a supportive relationship with Penny's mother.

Procrastinating as long as I could, I called Paula Thursday night. I told her I had a sick kid in the hospital; I said I was sorry. What I didn't ask was whether I might come up to Philadelphia in a week or two.

Paula might have been the perfect person to share not just Penny but the whole goddamn 2 East experience with. But I wasn't very good at sharing. In reality, I didn't share my feelings with anyone.

• • •

On Friday morning, Penny's blood culture was positive: *Staph. aureus.* Penny continued to eat but at a slower pace. She was moderately defiant when I examined her, and whether she liked it or not, she was examined twice in the morning and afternoon.

When Jerry asked me about weekend care of Penny, I told him I had canceled my trip. He raised his eyebrows in a perplexed expression that quickly turned solemn. "I wish I could say I don't understand, but I do."

"Thanks." I appreciated my comrade not berating me. "As I recall, you were in and out of here all day on a Saturday in late December," I added.

"Yeah, that was for Samuel," he said, "and I would have been in and out on Sunday as well, but he died Saturday night. Let me know if there's anything I can do, Ben."

An exam Friday evening suggested Penny was holding her own, so I went home.

Saturday morning, Morgan informed me Penny was still eating but not with her usual vigor. She put up very little resistance when I examined her. Bad news. The sensitivities of the staph, isolated from Penny's blood culture, demonstrated only weak or no inhibition of the bacterial growth to a panel of antibiotics.

Jerry got me out of the Clinical Center for lunch. We didn't mope over our patients; we may have talked about what we were going to do the following year.

During the day, Penny's condition declined. She was less responsive, and at a quarter past seven, I wrote that she was now semicomatose. The blood bank was holding both packed red blood cells and platelets for Penny, in case I thought one or both might help. Penny was in remission, I reminded myself. I decided to spend the night on 2 East.

"Doctor Humphrey, there's nothing you can do. Go home," Barbara protested. "We take care of sick kids, not sick doctors."

Barbara was a seasoned veteran of very sick kids and someone I respected. I knew that there was nothing I could do, but I didn't want to drive back to Kirkhill. I didn't think I could sleep at home, so I stayed on 2 East.

I was falling in and out of sleep on a sofa in the waiting room when Barbara brought me a blanket and in a pseudogruff manner said, "Well, I guess we can take care of sick doctors too."

Sunday morning, stupor had given way to coma, and Penny did not respond when I examined her.

Rick came in to see one of his kids. I went over Penny's orders with him. He couldn't think of anything else to do. If there had been anything else, I was sure Barbara would have brought it to my attention. I asked about switching to different antibiotics.

"Why not," he said. "She's gone downhill on the combination you have her on. Too bad we can't order a white-blood-cell transfusion."

Sunday dragged on; the change in antibiotics didn't seem to make a difference. I decided to spend another night.

Then, on Monday at two in the morning, Barbara ran into the waiting room and shouted, "Penny just bit a nurse!"

"Yes!" I was happy at this misfortune for some poor nurse. Penny's eyes were open—not wide but open.

I drove home in the dark. Fresh air through the open windows invigorated me. It wasn't that I had saved Penny; I had been there when she exerted her will to live.

It was great to be alive.

• • •

At Kirkhill, I tried to be quiet, but Frank was awake and asked, "Are you OK?"

I said yes, almost shouting, and he looked at me as if to say, "How in the hell can you be excited at three in the morning?"

After sunrise, I smelled fresh coffee and enjoyed the warmth of a shower and the feel of clean clothes. Already at work, Frank had left me a note, telling me he fed the horses. Still, I wanted to see them, listen to them nicker and watch them charge the fence. We were out of carrots, so I gave them some sweet feed.

At 10:05 a.m., I walked into the doctors' office. Before I could greet Jerry, I saw that look on his face.

"Ben, Penny died this morning at 7:30 a.m. There was nothing you could have done, so we let you sleep. Dee and the nurses took care of all of the details. I'm sorry."

I told Jerry I was going for a short walk. I went to my bench, alone. I missed my buddy Squirrel. I had lost Penny; I lacked the insight to realize I had also lost Paula.

• • •

"Let's get a cup of coffee. I haven't seen you for a couple of weeks," Myron said.

"I've been embarrassed about being one of the bad boys last year," I said, hanging my head. "You know, protocol violations. I know it was wrong; I feel bad about it."

"There haven't been any recent protocol violations," Myron said. "Tom Frei and Jay Freireich never mentioned your delaying therapy, and all three of you guys are known to take good care of your patients. I sit in on the weekly review of the chemotherapy trials."

I nodded. I knew that none of us would ever do that again. Still, I wanted his input on things. "Myron, it's hard not to fall in love with these kids; you want to protect 'em. Contrary to my training and all of my role models in internal medicine, I've been and I remain emotionally involved with my patients. I just lost a little girl, a two year old."

"Penny Tapley, I know," Myron said. "I remember my own training. It's okay to care for 'em, worry about 'em, fall in love with 'em, but when you sit down to write orders, on 2 East you're a physician. You're trying to prolong remissions, trying to cure 'em." His look was pensive, and I knew Myron understood how tough it was: putting kids like Penny through the hell of POMP therapy, knowing that toxicity might follow.

I shrugged and nodded. It seemed like a good formulation. I regretted our missteps in the fall, and I was committed to staying the course with the POMP protocol. Last Monday when Penny's marrow was hypoplastic, it didn't cross my mind to delay therapy but it evoked some emotional turmoil.

"You know, Ben," Myron said, "we come out of our training young, idealistic, and immature. 2 East is a place where guys like you can grow up. We don't go into medicine to cause the pain that's induced by marrow aspirations or the suffering associated with toxicity. But we don't go into research to perpetuate the status quo. We're going to cure this disease, Ben. We can talk about it further over coffee. Come on."

Part III:
Coming-of-Age

MARCH

O n the first day of March, I walked out of the cottage and greeted the morning. The horses were at the fence, and the pasture was a velvet green of young grass-blades that pierced the air, scenting a warm breeze with the aroma of fertile earth. Wow, Humphrey, it's been a while since you indulged in such romantic imagery! Start your morning at the fence; be refreshed by the husbandry of feeding your equine friends. There were reasons to look forward to the day. I liked caring for my children and listening to their mothers, and you never knew when there might be a teddy bear needing examination. Stop whining about being an internist on a pediatric floor, and just enjoy being a physician.

• • •

G ood news: all of my children were in remission. Nice way to start the month. Warmer weather meant I would take a sandwich and coffee out to my bench at NIH. I was joined for the first time by a young squirrel, red coat, bushy tail, and all. I wondered if he was a son of my buddy Squirrel. Why not assume so? Time again for me to invest in peanuts and a new lunch companion.

After work, I started a new routine. After changing into jeans, a sweatshirt, and tennis shoes, I caught Domino, grabbed a handful of his thick mane, and jumped onto his broad back. The evening was cool, but the body heat from Domino's broad, fat back radiated through my jeans and warmed my legs. I got a short ride, and Domino got an extra handful of sweet feed. A surefire way to enjoy Kirkhill.

• • •

On Tuesday morning, Dee greeted me with a smile. "You have a new admission, Doctor Humphrey. Hilary O'Keefe is four years old. She's from Ireland. You're going to like her. She's a real charmer."

Then Dee frowned. "Her father's a pathologist and has just joined the staff here at NIH. The family elected to travel by boat, and Hilary's leukemia became clinically evident during the voyage."

Hilary sat on her mother's lap, shy, leaning back onto her mother's chest, flanked by a brother on each side. The body language was clear: "Don't hurt our sister." It was a striking image.

The younger boy, probably five or six, was the casual one. Sheaves of sandy hair were stacked in a random manner over a smooth forehead, and his blue shirt was mostly tucked into his brown shorts, but his socks were up and both shoes properly tied. He was leaning ever so slightly against his mother.

The older brother stood on his own. His brown hair was parted to one side and neatly combed, his eyes peering out from a long face, observing my every move. Pants, shirt, and shoes all matched in shades of brown.

I started with the younger. "I'm Doctor Humphrey. What's your name?"

"Brendan." A slight smile.

I told him I would be one of the doctors taking care of Hilary and then asked, "In Ireland, do you guys give each other five?" I held out my hand. He didn't know. So I demonstrated. Then, whack—a good smack. "Yeah," I said with a little body language, "good one!"

Turning to the older brother, I asked his name.

"I'm Liam." There was no smile.

Holding out my hand, I got a pro-forma five back.

"Hi, Hilary. I'm Doctor Humphrey," I said, holding out my hand.

Slowly, she placed the tips of four fingers onto my open palm, looked at her fingers on my hand and then at me, turned her head a little, and smiled. She was pale, her abdomen slightly swollen. Despite a peaked look, she had a beautiful, full face; her soft short brown hair had been curled. There were ecchymoses on both forearms but no petechiae.

"It's been kind of tough week, hasn't it, Hilary?"

With that she turned her head toward her mother and smiled. All children are endearing, but some are enchanting.

Mrs. O'Keefe gave Hilary a little hug and rested her cheek on her head.

"I'm going to ask your mother a few questions about your sister: how long she's been sick, what was done—you know, so on and so forth. Would that be OK?" I asked, looking at the two brothers.

Brendan nodded and smiled, and Liam almost nodded, his stiffness softened.

In her early thirties, Mrs. O'Keefe was articulate, her voice suggesting an Irish accent.

"She had a real bad bloody nose," Brendan volunteered.

"That's right," Mrs. O'Keefe said, looking at Brendan. "On the second day out."

"Hilary got blood all over one of my books," Brendan added.

"We took her to the sick bay; the ship's doctor and my husband found that Hilary had an enlarged spleen and liver."

"I held a wet washcloth over her nose," Liam said with some pride, wanting to contribute.

"They looked at Hilary's blood under the microscope. It was leukemia. My husband is a pathologist." Tears rolled down Mrs. O'Keefe's cheeks. Brendan patted his mother's arm, and Liam put his hand on her shoulder. She did not apologize for crying and accepted the support of her sons, enfolding her daughter in a cradle of care.

This was not only a disease of the bone marrow; it was a blow to the entire family.

• • •

While I explained the status of Hilary's marrow, Doctor O'Keefe entered the room. He apologized for being late, as he'd stayed in their rented home to receive some of the family's property arriving from Ireland. He introduced himself as James O'Keefe, and I was pleased to know his first name wasn't Doctor. He walked over to Hilary, took her hand and spoke to her, then turned to his wife, and ended by assuring both his sons that everything was going to be all right. There was something very warm about the way he interacted with his family. He addressed me as Doctor Humphrey and said Doctor Freireich had informed him I would be caring for Hilary.

When I offered to make a copy of the POMP protocol, he declined. "I'd be happy to take you up to the lab to look at Hilary's marrow," I said.

Declining again and thanking me, Doctor O'Keefe said, "I'm just Hilary's father. You and Doctor Freireich are her doctors."

Being Hilary's physician, I thought, would be a real pleasure, and she had two great brothers. This was going to be a new pattern; all new admissions would be an opportunity to get to know yet another child.

• • •

A nervous father-to-be, Rick kept us up to date on all his patients. If he had to leave in the middle of the day or couldn't make rounds the next day because Jody went into labor, there wouldn't be any problem with coverage of his children. Jerry and I made rounds with Rick in the morning and in the late afternoon, so after a few days we knew Rick's children and their moms almost as well as our own charges.

• • •

O n March 10, when I walked into the nurses' station, I was greeted by, "Doctor H.! It's a boy, a healthy baby boy, eight pounds, four ounces. Jody's fine. They're going to call him Erik," Morgan said, sticking her head out of the medication room. Brigid, sitting by a stack of charts, looked up with a big smile.

I'd go see my half of Rick's children and tell their mothers the good news. As I walked out of the nurses' station, I was greeted by Dee, who in joyous tones repeated the good news.

When I entered Rick's dying seven-year-old Susan Stevens's room, Mrs. Stevens said, "We were expecting you, Doctor Humphrey. We heard about Erik."

Weak from anemia, Susan managed a smile and said, "A newborn baby."

So it went as I continued my rounds on Rick's children. One of Rick's six-year-olds, Alice, wanted to know if I had a baby. When I told her no, she frowned and pursed her lips. Whether Alice's response was disapproval or sadness, I didn't know, but I felt bad at disappointing her with my answer.

This was a bad-news floor, so the birth of a baby reverberated throughout as if some golden bell had been brought out of storage and rung for the first time.

Last summer I'd asked Rick, "What's the worst part of being a resident in pediatrics?"

"Being called into the delivery room to be on standby as a pediatrician for a high-risk delivery, a very old or very young mother, or a fetus with slow heart rate just before birth, et cetera."

Later in the year, Jerry asked, "You want a son or a daughter?"

G. Bennett Humphrey

"I just want a healthy baby and no complications for Jody."

Jody was young and healthy, and Rick's anxiety had passed. I wondered if we should issue Erik a banjo.

• • •

Before I met Jon Pope for the first time, Rick had told me in private that Jon was extremely ward wise, with a unique capacity to look at reality. Rick said he had talked to a lot of kids in Minnesota who were critically ill or dying, but Jon was in a class of his own, a very courageous kid. "Let me tell you what Jon said when I told him he had relapsed last month: 'The monthly bone marrow aspiration, if good, same old chemotherapy. Relapse; new drugs, new toxicity. Green sign on the door: *Oxygen in Use* Sigh up, a very sick kid. Sign gone: a dead kid.

'I just nodded. Both Rick and I understood that all the children on 2 East knew about the green sign; even toddlers who could not yet read knew that oxygen was for very sick kids. When a green sign was up, traffic by that door increased. They tried to peek inside: a crying mother was a really bad sign.'"

During the three days that I made rounds with Rick before Eric was born, I had gotten to watch Jon in action. He was twelve, bright and observant, and liked to pull Rick's chain. When Rick explained that I would be taking over when his wife delivered, Jon said, "I assume Doctor Humphrey is better at starting IVs."

I couldn't let the remark pass, so I told Jon, "My hands tremble—sometimes."

Jon quipped, "That's OK. Doctor Lottsfeldt passes out when he sees blood."

On the first day I took over Jon's care, I was greeted by Morgan. "Jon's IV has infiltrated, Doctor Humphrey. I've packed his arms in hot towels, and it should be relatively easy to find a vein."

254

Breaking Little Bones

The IV was started on the first stick, and when I finished, Jon was ready. "That's not the best IV I've ever had started on me." Jon wore a small smile. "This was your first one, right?" The smile broadened. "You'll get better, Doc."

I returned the smile, respecting this no-BS doctor-patient relationship, but inside I didn't feel very good. Jon had been in remission for six months on POMP and then relapsed last month and received daunomycin. Yesterday, a blood culture grew out a gram-negative rod that this morning was identified as *E. coli.* IV antibiotics were already started. Jon had a lot of spunk, but he was critically ill.

"Take me into the hall," Jon implored the next morning.

"You're kind of weak," I said. I got a wheelchair and IV pole. He looked neither up nor down the hall but at his door: room number, his name, and nothing more.

If having your hand taped to an IV board and a needle inserted into your arm was the sacrament of the anointing of the sick, the green sign on your hospital door was the same thing as your last rites.

On the third day, Jon aroused himself as I listened to his chest. He focused his strength to say, "Hall."

Brigid had to help me get Jon into the wheelchair. Out into the hall for a look at his door and then back to bed.

There was something noble about Jon and something sterile about the note I wrote that morning in his chart. *Bone-marrow failure, neutropenia. Progressive* E. coli *sepsis, found this morning to be semicomatose. Jon's condition reclassified from seriously ill to critical.*

We never hung a green sign, but late in the afternoon of that third day, we took his name off the door.

• • •

On the upper-right-hand corner of my desk was a note: "Carl Shively: Should he stay on 6-MP, or should Rx be D/C? Discuss further therapy for the next year with Doctor Friereich in March."

The VAMP, BIKE, and POMP protocols included a date for the cessation of therapy, but this older daily 6-MP schedule did not.

I asked Rick if there were any long-term survivors being followed at the University of Minnesota, and he told me no. The librarian helped me with a literature search on stopping therapy in long-term survivors: nothing helpful. The medical-records office pulled Carl's chart; I reviewed it again, especially the letters from other centers. Giving the record to Jay's secretary, I asked if I could see him the next day to discuss Carl's therapy.

"Come in, Ben. It's about the Shively kid, isn't it?" Jay said in a pleasant manner, looking up from a pile of other charts.

"There has been no evidence of leukemia in his peripheral blood or his bone-marrow aspirates for four years," I reported. "His mother is not pushing for either continuing or discontinuing the 6-mercaptopurine. The question is what you want me to do."

"I don't care what you do," Freireich said with a shrug.

"What do you mean? I don't know what to do. I've been on 2 East for nine months, and you've been directing 2 East for ten years. Don't you have some preference?"

"This is one time when experience is of no value. You're a doctor; you're his doctor; make a decision. No one has any experience managing patients in long-term remission with 6-MP. Secondly, what you do tomorrow will not contribute to the cure of leukemia. Grow up. I am not here to ease your feelings. This is a research institute." Jay stared at me with a neutral expression.

Another goddamn lesson in growing up. Take responsibility. You can't spend the rest of your life with someone holding your hand.

Disappointment or frustration must have swept across my face because Jay continued, "Look, Ben, there's nothing I can learn from your patient Shively that's going to help me write the next protocol for leukemia. He's a fluke. I don't even know if daily oral 6-MP represents a three percent cure rate. I'd have to put a couple hundred patients on that 6-MP regimen to find out if there's another kid like Shively. I told all three of you that we're looking for a ten to twenty percent or greater cure rate."

It took Jay long enough to say all of that for me to calm down. Dammit, I thought. He's right again. But I wasn't trained to think in these terms. If I had a problem, I went to the library or talked to someone who had more experience. Then I'd take the recommendation from a published article on the subject or someone's advice and do what seemed best.

"OK," I said. "I'll take responsibility for making a decision, but I'll be goddamned if I'm going to flip a coin. Five-year disease-free survival is often used to define a surgical cure. It may be irrelevant in leukemia. I'll tell Mrs. Shively that's the plan for now. If we learn something during this next year, we may stop earlier or treat for longer." I didn't look to Jay for approval and turned to leave.

"Now that wasn't so difficult, was it?" Jay said and went back to his pile of charts.

Being polite by nature, I said, "Thank you." That was appropriate. If I had been asked that question a few minutes earlier, I would have wanted to say, "You're a pain in the ass, Jay." To my surprise, I said, "Growing up is a pain in the ass."

On the way home to Kirkhill, I stopped and bought carrots. The horses got three each, and I spent extra time at the fence. My growth experience wasn't over. What was still bothering me, and what Jay hadn't thrown in my face, was the simple fact that I didn't want to be responsible if something went wrong. I wanted to be able to say, "We did what Jay thought best." But nobody knew what was best. I was going to do what I thought reasonable.

• • •

While I always enjoyed seeing Mrs. Shively and Carl, there was an extra dimension to seeing this boy in March. He was a symbol of what might be possible in treating leukemia. As viewed from 2 East in 1965, childhood leukemia was always a fatal disease. I had told Rick and Jerry about Carl. Assuming all went well today, I was planning on asking Mrs. Shively to visit the nurses on 2 East.

Mrs. Shively and Carl entered the exam room. "Sorry we're a bit late." Her demeanor was subdued. If Carl's therapy was a stressor for me, God only knew what she had been through during the last few weeks. Carl was my patient; he was her son.

After reassuring Mrs. Shively, I said to Carl, "Let's get this bone marrow out of the way." As usual, I took the bone marrow up to pathology, waiting impatiently for the elevator. Up in the path lab, I watched the technologist process the smears. Each step was timed and only took a minute or two, but it seemed like forever. Finally, looking down into the microscope, I saw a beautiful remission marrow.

Returning to the clinic, I said, "Carl, your marrow is great. I mean, there's no leukemia. I'm going to continue the 6-MP for another year."

"Thank God. Oh, thank God." Mrs. Shively sobbed and blew her nose as dammed-up tears flooded her cheeks. "If you had said we were going to stop the 6-MP, we would have stopped. But I'm so glad you think it should be continued. "

"You know that as research continues, we may learn what constitutes a true cure, when we can stop maintenance therapy. When—"

"I know about research, Doctor Humphrey: the pain, the uncertainly, the waiting for the results of the bone marrow, the fear that your child is going…" She stopped.

Carl embraced his mother. "Everything's OK, Mom."

The bravado returned. "This discussion of stopping therapy did the whole family a world of good. A real catharsis. Carl's dad and I have had a lot of great talks. We want to make a small donation to the clinic. To whom do I make the check out?"

Calling Jay's office, I was told he'd be glad to see Mrs. Shively. I told Carl, "Go shake Doctor Freireich's hand; he's been directing research here on leukemia for ten long and difficult years. He needs to see, listen to, and experience your good health."

"Mrs. Shively, if I may make a suggestion, tell Doctor Freireich that you and Carl's dad would like the donation to be earmarked for the nurses of 2 East, to buy anything they need for the children that they can't get out of the NIH budget. Then stop by Dee's office on 2 East and say hello. I'll be in the doctors' office if you want to tell me about your visit."

Thirty minutes later, a timid knock on the door. Mrs. Shively was agitated. "Oh, Doctor Humphrey, I was so nervous! I just lost it. I told Doctor Freireich I didn't think you guys knew what you were doing and I didn't care because I had Carl. It just came out, and you know what? He laughed, laughed out loud. It was the wrong thing to say. I apologized, but he said it was OK."

I laughed until I had to wipe a few tears away. "It was the right thing to say, and Doctor Emil J. Freireich has a sense of perspective. He's tough. He's honest, and he's dedicated."

"This is the first time I've been on 2 East since Carl's first and only hospitalization. I wanted to thank the nurses for the good care they gave Carl and their support for me. I didn't know if I should have taken them away from their work. They're so busy, but they were really glad to see Carl; they fussed over him and wanted to see him again."

"They need that, Mrs. Shively. We all need to see Carl. Give me five, guy."

After a resounding whack, he and his mother left.

My phone rang: "Ben, this is Jay. Thanks."

• • •

After a week of paternity leave, Rick returned to care for Susan Stevens, who was now comatose. When a child was really sick, the traffic pattern in the hall changed. Rather than going to the playroom, the kids walked by the sick child's room.

Jerry asked Rick, "Did you see this in Minnesota?"

"No. The pediatric wing was segregated by age, not disease."

I asked, "Which type of floor do you prefer?"

"This is the first time I've worked on a cancer ward, but I like it. It's a bummer on 2 East when a child is sick, but when no one is dying, it's better for the children; everybody is bald, everybody has an IV running, and almost everybody vomits."

"What about for you as a pediatric oncologist?" Jerry asked. "You're now working with two internists. No other pediatricians to discuss problems with."

"I relate better with you two guys than I ever have with fellow pediatric house officers. There's no petty jealousness or one-upmanship." Rick paused. "It has nothing to do with your being internists. I get the kind of support I need."

"That works both ways," Jerry said.

I nodded in agreement.

• • •

I realized how much I enjoyed seeing each of my children at the beginning of their monthly visits—that is, before I had to do the marrow and start an IV. I could see from their height and weight that they were growing, but the biggest difference was their manner of greeting and the verbal games or conversations we had the rest of the week. One could observe and take joy in their growth and development.

On the third Monday of the month, Mrs. Sullivan and Billy came down the hall. Walking directly up to me, Billy extended his right hand and said, "Good morning, Doctor Humphrey."

Switching a chart out of my right hand, I shook Billy's hand. "Good morning, Billy. How are you?"

Looking at his mother for recognition of this accomplishment, Billy was rewarded with a smile and nod of approval. Saying something about the playroom, Billy scooted down the hall.

Mrs. Sullivan explained that his dad had taught him to shake hands.

"He's no longer a toddler; he's a little boy. I only see Billy for part of a week each month; maybe the changes are more striking to me. By the way, where's Bear?"

"Billy has formed a friendship with another boy from his preschool class," Mrs. Sullivan explained. "Billy abandoned Bear, but I rescued him and dusted him off, and now he has an honored place on a bookshelf in our study."

The story of Bear transported me back to the late spring of 1963. I was about to share that moment with Billy's mom when I caught myself. I told her we'd do the marrow right away.

Finishing my chores for the morning, grateful that Billy's bone marrow was leukemia-free, I went out to my bench to see my little friend, deciding to call him Son of Squirrel. He too was developing; he had learned to sit on his haunches, looking cute. He got his peanuts while I remembered that moment in the spring of 1963. During WFMT's *The Midnight Special*, they played a new song by Peter, Paul and Mary: "Puff, the Magic Dragon." The song enchanted me, but one line leaped out: "A dragon lives forever but not so little boys."

• • •

One afternoon, Mrs. Yardley called. She told me she wanted to come back to 2 East. "Just to walk through. I want my husband to see the nursing unit."

I said they would be welcome anytime and that I would like to meet Todd's dad; I remembered the day he called, the day that Todd died after falling down the stairs and hitting his head.

Mrs. Yardley was still trying to adjust but doing better.

"How's Ralph?"

"Well," she said, "Ralph moped around the house for over a month; I guess we moped together, but he's recovered. He's now constantly at my side, and you won't believe this, Doctor Humphrey, but I talk to him just like Todd used to. He's always there for me."

"I believe you," I said. "I talk to a squirrel, three horses, and a black lab myself."

• • •

Time moved on. I didn't need to mark the halfway point of the month. Kirkhill was still an enjoyable break, but it wasn't a respite between courses of POMP.

The last Saturday morning of March, all my emotions were in the moment. While I was filling the horses' watering trough, a bird warbled in the tree between the fence and the barn. In the west, the tips of Shenandoah Mountain's peaks could be seen on the far horizon. Frank had planted a floral display of red, yellow, and purple pansies in front of the cabin. Bees flew among the flowers, a sure sign of spring.

I thought of Henry Reed's poem "Naming of Part," in which the voice of the drill instructor explaining the parts of the rifle is set in contrast to the thoughts of a recruit. I particularly liked the last two stanzas:

> *And this you can see is the bolt. The purpose*
> *Is to open the breech, as you see. We can slide it*
> *Rapidly backwards and forwards: we call this*
> *Easing the spring. And rapidly backwards and forwards*
> *The early bees are assaulting and fumbling flowers:*
> > *They call it easing the Spring.*
>
> *They call it easing the Spring: it is perfectly easy*
> *If you have any strength in your thumb: like the bolt,*
> *And the breech, and the cocking-piece, and the point of balance,*
> *Which in our case we have not got; and the almond-blossom,*
> *Silent in all of the gardens and the bees going backwards and forwards,*
> > *For to-day we have naming of parts.*

Closing the book, I thought, it's nice to have friends who are poets when you're hungry for the right words, but I also need breakfast. I put a scrambled egg and some bacon between two slices of toast and went back to the fence.

Sitting under the tree in front of the barn, I reflected on the pace of things on 2 East. I had started in July as a beast of burden resenting this year as being of little value to my career—a year not part of my plan. I reflected on the previous year in Germany. If I were honest, that year wasn't of great academic value either, but it was an investment in learning about another culture, another way of life. Germany was a romantic adventure to be retrieved in the future, when I might question if life itself was worthwhile. Now, on 2 East I had experienced the love of children who forgave me for the needles I used and shared their world with me. The children were honest, from Sarah Thompkins's hostility to Sally Carter's hugs. The camaraderie of Jerry and Rick was powerful, as was the respect I was experiencing in watching and listening to the mothers and the nurses of 2 East. And then there was Freireich.

APRIL

Three more months of Monday mornings. The joy of exchanging a smile or feeling a hug, the sinking feeling on hearing, "We're ready for you in the treatment room," the breaking of a little bone, the little ones with their arms up, indicating they wanted to be carried back to their room, the warmth of a small body against my chest and arms around my neck, the absolution of a head resting on my shoulder, the impatience of waiting to look down the microscope, the sigh of relief upon seeing normal cells, and the delight of telling that to the mother—all these emotions went with the yin and yang of bone-marrow aspiration. And I asked myself, would you really rather be up on 12 East doing this procedure on adults?

• • •

After the screaming, the week ran smoothly. There was black ink on the Board, and it was as if someone had stolen the red marker, and all the children went home on Friday afternoon. Sign-out rounds at noon on Friday were over in less than five minutes. Then, the two bachelors listened as Rick divulge the delights of fatherhood.

• • •

That first Saturday morning started with a cold, wet nose: Shonto was on the wrong side of the front door. Enough of dawn resounded through the bedroom window to inform me it was time to get up. I followed a wagging tail to the front door, let her out, and stood outside our cabin door. Calm air celebrated the placid nature of Kirkhill, and morning sunlight on a western ridge called me to the fence. A soaring mourning dove ruffled the air.

Shonto raised her ears to a bark from across the pasture, and she piped a tracheal response. I chuckled. "Well done, Shonto. I liked your canine pastorale." The dog in the drinking-water game followed.

Frank had said it very well: Kirkhill is a modern cabin by Walden. We didn't have a pond, but we had a water trough for the horses.

• • •

Looking at the Board on Monday, I smiled. Hilary, my Irish rose, was to be admitted for POMP. Other than a marrow aspirate and an IV, it should be a pleasant week. There would also be Mrs. O'Keefe and Hilary's brothers, Liam and Brendan.

Walking into Hilary's room, I noted that neither brother was flanking Hilary. Brendan was busy with a book. Despite her loss of hair, Hilary was still pretty. Liam was relaxed, but he had a black eye. I said hello to Hilary, greeted her mother, and started with Brendan, who gave me a good hard five. Liam actually smiled.

"Well, Liam, what happened to you?"

"That's a shiner," Brendan said.

Mrs. O'Keefe said, "A neighborhood boy started to make fun of Hilary's baldness, and Liam came to her defense."

"I wasn't there, or I would have helped," Brendan said, swinging a fist.

"I would have beaten him up, if Ma hadn't gotten in the way." Liam looked at his mother. "I know, I know. We're not supposed to fight."

Charming as usual, Hilary told me that, in the future, she was going to wear her wig when they went out. We talked about wigs being hot and how Maryland could be very warm in the summer. Apparently, her parents had prepared her for the hair loss. "Hilary told me she was now just like all the other kids on 2 East," Mrs. O'Keefe said.

A good week could be anticipated, because Hilary was in remission. Her counts weren't too low, so a fever might not occur. During the week, I told Hilary about cycling around Dublin the previous summer and the time I rode my bike the wrong way on a one-way street and was stopped by a policeman. He was very stern and unfriendly until he heard my American accent. When he found out I was from Chicago, he wanted to know if I knew his cousin Sean Murphy, who also lived in Chicago. Hilary and Brendan laughed.

When I commented that, because of my budget, all I ate was fish-and-chips or mixed grill, Liam interrupted, "Yuck! Nobody should have to eat mixed grill!"

Brendan wanted to join the conversation. "I like fish-and-chips."

The two brothers then described their likes and dislikes of Irish food. I told Brendan that true fish-and-chips weren't commonly available here in the United States, and I told Liam that mixed grill wasn't available at all.

One day when Hilary and her two brothers were in the playroom, I told Mrs. O'Keefe a tale Rick had shared. He was caring for a young boy with leukemia from a small town in Minnesota. His older, stronger, and tougher brother found out his younger brother was being teased, so he had his head shaved. That put an end to it, and being bald was thereafter popular. I'd elected not to tell that story in front of Hilary's brothers.

"Well, if one of them wants to have his head shaved, we'll let him do that. All three can be at each other's throats at home, but the boys have always been very protective of Hilary out on the street."

A tolerant mother, two protective brothers, and an enchanting little girl—a well-tempered quartet.

● ● ●

Breaking Little Bones

O n our desks one morning in April was a notice from Jay:

> Protected Environment
> Demonstration of the Life Island
> Wednesday 12 April at 1300 hours
> Conference Room 12 East
> Required attendance: Clinical Associates
> of 2 East and 12 East.
> *Emil J. Freireich, MD*

"One o'clock," Jerry said. "That means no free lunch." He was in a bad mood; he had just lost an eight-year-old. "Another sacrifice on the LD10 altar."

That afternoon, we rode the elevator together. In the conference room was the so-called Life Island: a hospital bed enclosed in a plastic canopy. At the foot of the bed, a stainless-steel box or console stood five feet tall, a foot or two wider than the bed, and three feet thick. The air intake was on the lower third of the console. The purr of electrical motors pumped filtered air into the inflated canopy. Clear plastic double doors on the upper third of the metal box served to transfer food into and waste out of the Island.

Unlike the panther's cage in the zoo, there was no room for a padded gait back and forth even the length of the bed. I was remembering Rilke's "Der Panther." Someone in a business suit made some remarks. A nurse demonstrated the ports on each side, their long sleeves and gloves allowing nurses to change sheets and physicians to start IVs or draw blood.

Freireich began. "Fatal infections are a limiting factor on how much chemotherapy can be given. This unit will allow greater doses and more days of therapy."

"How much more therapy, Jay?" Rick asked.

"The dose of each drug in POMP will be doubled. The drugs will be infused for ten days rather than five."

Absolute silence filled the room. Then Jerry muttered, "An LD50, if not higher."

Freireich fractured the icy air: "We will start with a young adult. Before the patient enters the unit, the skin will be cleansed with surgical soap and the bowel cleaned out with nonabsorbable antibiotics. There will be round-the-clock nursing coverage, and clinical associates from both 12 and 2 East will also help. Any problem, large or small, call me in my office or at home."

"What are the criteria for immediately removing the patient from the unit without waiting for your approval?" Jerry asked.

Jay shook his head and said, "No reason or need for that."

Jerry persisted, "If the patient slashed his wrist?"

The business suit jumped up. "We've spent time and money on the psychiatric profiles of patients who can adapt to this environment." He added with pride, "I have personally spent several days in the Life Island."

Jerry looked around. Blank faces—no one cared.

Riding down in the elevator, Rick sighed. "At least it's not on 2 East. Can you imagine a kid in that unit?"

I thought out loud. "Plastic walls are as good as bars."

Jerry said, "I like that."

I said, "It's not original but a paraphrase from Rilke. I'll bring the poem in tomorrow."

The next morning, Jerry read in silence. "I like it. Rick, listen to this. It's a poem called 'The Panther.'" He read out loud, "'His vision from the passing of the bar / is grown so weary that it holds no more. / To him it seems there are a thousand bars / and behind a thousand bars no world.'"

• • •

In the early evening, Rick and I were in the nurses' station writing notes on a series of admissions. The phone rang: "It's 12 East. The young man in the Life Island is threatening to break out, and there's no physician on the floor," Barbara said.

"You're the internist, Ben," Rick said with a giggle. We all knew a twenty-year-old undergraduate with leukemia had been entombed in the Life Island seven days ago. After getting on the elevator, I wondered, what am I going to do? Patient selection based on psychiatric profile: that's got to be a bunch of bullshit. How could anybody predict the response of a young man to the stress of this ten-day double dose of POMP, coupled with the pseudo-isolation of a clear canopy and its lack of privacy? Solitary confinement was the ultimate threat in prison, and in this case it was confinement in a bubble so everybody could watch. The poor guy couldn't even scratch his balls without the nurse taking note.

"What's this young man's name?" I asked the nurse who met me halfway down the hall.

"Walter. We just gave him Seconal to calm him down. It's a standing order. He likes to be called Walt," she said, leading me down to the room.

Walt looked like a football player. He sat on the edge of the bed; if he wanted out, he could get out. Another nurse with an arm through a port, wearing a rubber glove, was holding his hand. Ah, I thought cynically, TLC rendered by a sterile hand.

Shooting from the hip, I started with, "It's gotta be hell in there, Walt."

"I just want to walk in the hall," he said.

I tried logic first, comments on trying to cure a bad disease…

Walt interrupted. "Can't you put me in a sterile surgical gown?"

Needing to buy time, I asked, "Where are you going to school, Walt?"

We spoke of college: the commitment, difficult courses, work for the future.

Walt persisted. "Just for a few minutes. Then I promise I'll crawl back in."

That ploy hadn't worked either. "Listen, Walt," I said with some frustration, "it's not impossible that, next year, we'll ask you to help us; ask you to stand on this side of the clear plastic curtain; ask you to help another patient to stay inside, to complete the therapy."

We exchanged a long stare; Walt's shoulders dropped, and he nodded, swung his feet around, and lay back down.

While I was writing my note in Walt's chart, Jay stuck his head into the nurses' station.

"What's going on?"

I replied that Walt would stay in the unit.

Jay went to check for himself. He returned and asked me, "What'd you tell him?" So I went over the sequence. Self-preservation and commitment hadn't worked, but altruism might have been of value.

"Good idea."

"Thanks, but it could have been the Seconal. What I said might have been totally unrelated."

A reflective calm swept across Freireich's face. "You're not going to take credit for convincing Walt to stay in the unit. You know, Ben, at times you have been critical of me. But you can think analytically and be critical of your own actions."

That night I thought, the Life Island seems like a dumb idea, but if Jay's going to make any progress for the future, he's got to use his imagination today. That's the long haul of a career in research.

During the next week, I should have inquired how Walt responded to the chemotherapy and what the result of all this effort was. I ought to have asked an associate from 12 East to keep me posted. I could have gone up to 12 East just to pay a social call, to see if Walt wanted to talk to someone who wasn't writing orders on his care. But I didn't do any of these things. My world was 2 East, and I hoped I'd never see one of those units on my floor.

• • •

"Let's go for coffee, Ben," Jerry said. Then with a thespian flair, he added, "Let us go then, you and I, / When the evening is spread out against the sky…"

When asked what that was from, Jerry said, "'The Love Song of J. Alfred Prufrock.' Poetry! I bought a collection of poems by Rilke. Good reading." Then he asked, "Did you major in literature as an undergraduate?"

"Heavens no," I said. "Remember I've got dyslexia?"

"But, Ben, I've noticed you know poetry and literature," Jerry said.

"Well, thanks, but my knowledge is limited to two sources. As a graduate student, I was in my laboratory every evening with an FM radio on my desk. The classical music station, WFMT, signed off each night with a poem. So during all those graduate-school years, I heard recordings of Elizabeth Bishop, Robert Frost, Dylan Thomas, and so on. A great way to end the day and a reminder to go home and get some sleep."

"Neat," Jerry said.

"The second source was Untermeyer's pocket anthology of poetry, which I read during ski trips and other outdoor adventures."

"Why aren't you more open about the role of poetry in your life?" Jerry asked.

"The University of Chicago was a great place for me, but it was full of eggheads. I once commented that I liked dogs and children, and a good friend in the humanities reminded me of W. C. Fields by quoting, 'A man who hates children and dogs can't be all bad.' So I was trained to be careful about sentimental interests."

"I get it. Romantics weren't taken seriously. Well, I don't agree. I majored in English as an undergraduate at Princeton." Then Jerry said with a chuckle, "You know, on rounds with Freireich, I often think it would be more relevant to quote a poem than a scientific article from *Cancer Research*. Jerry took a piece of paper, scribbled several lines and then read out loud. "You know, something like this: To-morrow, and to-morrow, and to-morrow, / Creeps in this petty POMP research pace / To its last line in the literature. / And all our yesterdays have led our kids / The way to dusty death. Out, out, brief candle! / You've strut and fret your hour upon 2 East / Your voices are heard no more. It is a tale / Told by no one, full of neutropenia and vomiting / Signifying everything."

I laughed and said, "Oh God, Jerry."

• • •

Two of my children were nearing the end of therapy and scheduled to stop POMP, so I asked Rick for help. "Well, I don't have any experience doing that," Rick said, "and I got a little fellow due to stop therapy in two months."

"But you've trained and worked with children and their mothers," I said. "You're also going to have to discuss stopping therapy in the next couple of months. You're obviously better prepared than Jerry or me."

"I'll say it again. Nothing prepares you for 2 East, Ben." Seeing a frown on my face, Rick continued. "Yeah, I've had a fellowship in pediatric hematology and oncology. During my two years at Minnesota, I followed lots of children, but they had a bunch of different problems. The diversity made things easier. Hematology is almost a vacation from oncology. Of course, children with sickle-cell anemia can have pain that's difficult to manage, but a child with hereditary spherocytosis—take the spleen out, and they're cured. Aplastic anemia—well, that can be fatal. Hemophilia is a bad chronic disease, but they rarely die on you."

"But you obviously treated children with cancer, didn't you?"

"The key word is *cancer*," Rick said. "There were lots of children with solid tumors, and some were cured with surgery, others were treated, and a few were cured with radiation therapy; most of the chemotherapy was oral or given in the outpatient department. And those with leukemia were never given POMP-type therapy. I'd go for months without a death."

I nodded.

"For those who don't relapse, they're going to have therapy discontinued because of the possibility of a cure. This cessation of therapy is mind-boggling to me, Ben."

In 1964, stopping therapy was the wave of the future. The three of us couldn't see it, but it was the beginning of the cure for childhood leukemia.

• • •

We asked Jay to discuss stopping therapy. "There are reasons to think that the previous protocols, called VAMP and BIKE, killed the residual leukemia cells in children. There are a few children from both of these protocols that are off therapy and remaining in remission. POMP is more intense, and I believe that fifteen months of therapy is enough."

Rick asked, "Do you think the cure rate might be ten percent?"

"I don't know. The number of kids off therapy is too small to calculate a number that can be believed," Jay explained. Seeing frustration on our faces, he slowed down. "Look, tell these mothers whose children are coming off therapy that there are theoretical considerations indicating we should stop. Tell 'em there are kids off therapy."

"Cell kinetics, theoretical considerations, someone else's child off therapy—I don't know if that's going to be meaningful for a mom who's looking at her son or daughter," Jerry said.

"All three of you guys have a reputation of spending time talking to your parents. Hold the line. You're not here to make things easy for them. You're not here to make parents happy. Your job is to follow the POMP protocol."

After Jay left, I said, "The POMP protocol. Our marching orders. But, you know, Jay didn't say POMP was God's gift to children with leukemia; he just said it was more intense. At least he's realistic and not one of those jerks who thinks he's on his way to Sweden."

Rick sat back in his chair. "We need to remember the hell Jay went through in developing platelet transfusion. There were those who didn't want him to try and those who wanted him to stop after a couple of early failures. The easy road would have been either not to try or to quit after the first two infusions. He persisted, and now we have platelets for transfusion."

Freireich was many things, but he was always honest. He was also tough; in his attack on leukemia, he wasn't trying to keep anyone happy.

• • •

Make an outline, Humphrey. An outline helps keep me from meaningless digression or using jargon as a smoke screen, I thought.

Sally Carter's mom made it clear last summer she was looking forward to the cessation of therapy, but Mrs. Thompkins had reservations about stopping therapy.

Some facts would be more relevant to one mom than to another, but they talked among themselves. So I'd better say the same thing to Mrs. Carter and Mrs. Thompkins. After a first draft, I made revisions by deleting some jargon and highlighted key points.

1. The *cessation* of therapy after fifteen months of treatment *is not an arbitrary decision.*
2. Experience with *real* children from 2 East had resulted in a few cases of long-term survival. Their chemotherapy had been stopped.
3. The therapy your child has been receiving is *more intense* than the previous protocols. Therefore, there should be more children who will achieve long-term remissions
4. Maybe the most compelling reason for stopping is *the risk of a life-threatening infection.* These deaths can occur in children in remission. That worries me every time Sally or Sarah returns for another course of POMP.

After reading the outline, I thought, God, I hate to approach these mothers with another reminder of the balance between chemotherapy preventions of relapse and therapy-induced toxicity.

"I understand, Doctor Humphrey," Mrs. Carter sighed. "I appreciate all that information. Thank you. It helps support our decision to stop. Close members of the family had discussed this on a few occasions. Sally's father and I have good support from these people."

Good old Mrs. Carter, I thought; she's trying to make my job easier. To my surprise, I told Mrs. Carter how fond I was of Sally. I hadn't planned on saying that—ad-lib comments weren't in my outline.

"I know that, and more importantly, Sally knows. You can't fool Sally. She talks about you; you're her Puzzle Doctor. And I think of you as the one who listens, Doctor Humpfee."

When I asked if she would be willing to talk to Mrs. Thompkins, Mrs. Carter said of course and that they had already discussed the matter a number of times.

Mr. and Mrs. Thompkins arrived on Monday. Sarah was scheduled to receive her last course of POMP. By chance, Brigid and I were standing in the hall as they entered. Mr. Thompkins was not physically imposing, despite a swagger to his gait. He was five ten or eleven, stocky, and wearing a stern persona. I suggested to the parents that we sit down in the doctors' office while Sarah was admitted. Brigid took Sarah to her room while I opened the door. Setting his shoulders, Mr. Thompkins walked boldly into the office, preceding his wife.

Mr. Thompkins listened impatiently to the first two points, shifting his weight from one haunch to the other. Then, before I started on point three, he said, "We have already decided to continue therapy. Doctor, you can't guarantee to me that my daughter will stay in remission if the drugs are stopped!"

I requested that he listen to the last two points. After I discussed the toxicity of POMP, I realized it was time to address Mr. Thompkins's question about a guarantee. I admitted that I couldn't forecast how Sarah would do. Then I paraphrased him: "Mr. Thompkins, you can't guarantee to me that a course of POMP in May won't kill your daughter!"

The persona of the man in charge was effaced by genuine frustration as he raised one eyebrow and sat up straight. "Are you telling me we have no choice? Are you saying I have to do what you say?" Mr. Thompkins shouted.

"No, Mr. Thompkins, I never said that." Sitting back in my chair and crossing my legs, I paused and let that sink in. "Sarah is your daughter, and you could have withdrawn her from this four-drug treatment schedule at any time during the last fifteen months, just as you can withdraw her from the schedule by taking her to another medical center where they can continue some sort of anticancer therapy." I paused.

Mr. Thompkins folded his arm across his chest.

"Let me give you an example of my concern about toxicity. Last July, Sarah spiked a fever at the end of a course of POMP. I had to keep her in the hospital and treat her for a potentially life-threatening infection. Your wife had to listen to Sarah cry, to deal with this threat to her life. Now, the fever wasn't due to bacteria, and Sarah went home. If Mrs. Thompkins had told me she didn't want to put her daughter through all that stress again, I would have asked her to think about it for the rest of the month before the next POMP was due. If she still wanted less intensive therapy, I would have made arrangements for that kind of therapy."

"But she didn't get that infection, and she hasn't had a problem since, Doctor," Mr. Thompkins growled as he pointed his index finger at me.

I almost asked him what he did for a living but thought, don't do that. It doesn't matter. He's the father, and you're the physician. How can you explain POMP or 2 East to a layman? If Rick wasn't prepared for 2 East - wait a minute. The moms know all about 2 East and all about POMP. Mrs. Thompkins hadn't said a word; get her into this exchange.

"Your wife knows about toxicity, Mr. Thompkins," I said. "She was here in July when a little girl named Jennifer Johnson—"

"It was so horrible, George!" she said, interrupting me. "I once tried to sit with Jennifer for a half an hour so her mother could go to lunch. I had to ask a nurse to come in. I couldn't do it." She accepted the tissues I handed to her.

Mr. Thompkins didn't care about my scientific reasons for stopping therapy, but he understood tears. "OK," he said to his wife.

"We'll think this over. I've got to get back to work."

When Mrs. Thompkins apologized for taking so much of my time, I assured her that I had plenty of time and admitted that this must be a difficult decision. I further suggested that we complete this last course of POMP and they think things over for the rest of the month. Out in the hall, Mr. Thompkins gave his wife a halfhearted hug and then headed for the exit, while she headed toward Sarah's room.

Walking out of the office, I noticed a handwritten note: "Dr. Humphrey is in conference." After pulling the sign off the door, I walked down to Dee's office and handed it to her.

"Are you still in one piece?" Dee smiled. "I knew Sarah's dad was upset. He was very rude to Brigid this morning when he called, demanding to see a doctor."

"If Mr. Thompkins wants to yell at me, that's OK—just part of my job. Being abrasive to a nurse wasn't OK. I'll personally tell him he was out of line, and he ought to apologize to Brigid."

"Please don't do that, Doctor Humphrey. We're professionals too."

I chuckled. "Touché."

• • •

Five of us were sitting in the cafeteria having coffee in the late afternoon: an associate from nephrology, another who was on the Metabolic Disease Service, a guy from cardiology, and Jerry and me.

The guy from cardiology wanted to know if any of us felt that the demands on our time were excessive.

The consensus was no. We were busy, but at the end of a day, we all felt we had completed our work. One could go to the library and even take an hour out for a sit-down lunch.

The associate from cardiology said he had spent more time talking to his patients during his first three months at NIH than during the entire three years of his residency in a large county hospital. "It's not like the good old days when I was unsupervised, overworked, and sleep-deprived, feeling that the best I could do was stopgap measures for patients I hardly knew," he said in a reflective tone.

"Well, I'm not overworked here—just bored. Give me the fast pace, the triage, the crisis management of an open ward in a county hospital. I don't get off talking to an alcoholic or some old bag lady," one of the other associates said.

The phrase *good old days* was an invitation for each of us to relate a favorite tale from residency. Like a reunion of seventy-year-old vets, we took turns telling our favorite war stories from the trenches of ward duty at a county or VA hospital. Truth wasn't important; embellishments for humor were the rules of engagement.

The cardiologist began. "At the county hospital where I trained, the disposition of a corpse was a despicable task. The body had to be wheeled to a freight elevator, taken to the basement, and pushed through a tunnel that connected the hospital to the county morgue in an adjacent building. This had to be done by a resident and couldn't be dumped on a medical student. The resident had to page a pathologist to accept the transfer of the body from the hospital to the morgue. There were forms to be filled out. It took time, and work piled up. Death on a ward was very unpopular." He smiled. "The guys working in the ER had an option. They would find out which ward had an open bed and leave a message with a nurse that a patient was being transferred. When some old codger died of a heart attack in the ER or in the waiting room, a brief admitting note was written with phony vital signs suggesting the patient was alive when leaving the ER, the body was thrown onto a gurney and taken in an elevator, and when the elevator doors opened onto the floor that had an empty bed, the body was pushed out into the hall, and the guys would run back to the ER and get back to work."

We were amused. His tale was believable.

The nephrologist cleared his throat. "I was once called by a surgical service as a consultant on an obese woman who was thought to be in renal failure. After a cholecystectomy, she had abdominal distension and no bowel sounds. The surgeons diagnosed paralytic ileus, and a long red Miller-Abbott tube was passed through her nose into the small bowel and hooked up to suction. That worked. Intestinal distension reduced, and normal bowel sounds returned, but she stopped making urine. It didn't make any sense. Because of the Miller-Abbot tube, she was receiving IV fluids, she wasn't gaining weight, and her kidney-function tests were normal. So I talked to the patient and asked if she peed when she sat on the bedpan. 'Oh yeah,' she told me, 'but the big red snake drinks it all.'"

We all laughed. The tale had been well told, but no one believed it. The Miller-Abbott tube is red, but it's only ten feet long, and the small intestine alone is twenty-two feet long.

The associate from the Metabolic Disease Service was next. "A patient was brought into an ER DOA because he bled to death after his penis had been cut off. A half an hour later, a woman known to have an uncontrolled-seizure disorder was admitted, also DOA. Her skull had been bashed in, and blood was coming out of her mouth. When they opened her mouth, they found a penis inside."

There were a few chuckles, but several of us said that tale had been attributed to county ERs in every large city. Whether that had ever happened didn't matter.

The cardiologist reflected and said, "I'm not sure I want to go back to that kind of ward medicine. This place has changed me. I enjoy talking to my patients, I like trying to answer their questions, and it's good to feel that you're working in a first-rate hospital."

They looked at me next. All my training had been at the hospitals and clinics of the University of Chicago. There were no wards. Patients were referred to specific members of the faculty from all over the Midwest. Good patient care was mandatory to keep that patient referral intact, but I wanted to contribute to the humor, so I turned to the cardiologist and said, "I agree with you. NIH does change you. I'm going to write a novel about this place."

"What are you going to call your novel, D-o-c-t-o-r Humphrey?" Jerry asked.

With a straight face, I quipped, "I Was a Pimp for POMP."

• • •

Polly Sorensen was admitted for her third monthly course of POMP. As on previous admissions, she wore her attire of gym shoes, blue denim overalls with a bib front, and a T-shirt. She was now completely bald and wore neither a scarf nor hat. She had achieved a remission with her first course, and with her second course, she seemed almost immune to toxicity. I knew she had some nausea, but she wasn't going to let that interfere with her socializing with the other kids on the floor. I began to think of Polly as my go-for-broke gal. She emitted energy as she greeted me and quickly dismissed any questions about toxicity and my inquiries into subtle signs or symptoms that might suggest a relapse. Polly just wasn't going to let POMP disrupt her life.

Mrs. Sorensen was as usual properly dressed for the season. She wore a full pink skirt and a white blouse, a pretty combination. She said that she and Polly wanted to talk to me about Polly keeping her head covered.

From the expression on Polly's face, I could tell it was Mom who wanted to discuss this topic, and Polly couldn't care less. I thought I had better move into this territory slowly. I didn't want to be used as leverage between this petite mom and her tomboy daughter. So I asked Mom what the issues were, and she said she wanted Polly to cover her head when out of the house. Polly had told her mother that cute little hats were a bother and wigs too warm.

I said they were both right. I turned my attention to Polly. After starting out with the fact that sunburn could be painful, I described secondary infection. I told Polly that the drugs she got here in the hospital weakened her ability to control infections. Shaking my head, I said, "The last thing you want to have to do is come back into the hospital for IV antibiotics—you know, an extra admission in between your scheduled monthly visits."

I was told emphatically, "No wig! No way!"

I told her all the kids said they were hot.

The expression on Mrs. Sorensen's face suggested she was satisfied with the conversation.

"OK, no wig," I said. "As I see it, there are three options: a baseball cap, a scarf, or a narrow-brimmed soft cotton hat. A scarf and a soft hat can be folded and stuffed into a pocket when you go back inside. Baseball caps are difficult to stuff into a pocket."

Polly's expression suggested she was pleased to have won on the wig but reluctant to yield on a scarf or hat. When I suggested there was a fourth possibility, she brightened up. I told her they made some very cute pink sun parasols, and before I could complete the sentence, Polly said no way. I quickly countered with, "How about a hat?"

"OK," Polly said. Looking at her mother, she asked, "Satisfied, Mom?" With that, she was out the door to visit Robert Thurman.

"Oh, Doctor Humphrey, I don't know what I'm going to do with her. She's such a tomboy," Mrs. Sorensen said. Noticing that I was laughing, she continued, "I don't think it's funny. I want a little girl, a daughter!"

I told her I wasn't laughing at Polly and certainly not at her but remembering my younger sister, who was a tomboy. When she was four and asked what she wanted for Christmas, she said she wanted a tin hat and a drum, and that was what she got. "Mrs. Sorensen, she turned out to be a pretty girl. A picture of her playing her cello and wearing a dress appeared on a national magazine, and she's now an attractive wife and mother. The tomboy years didn't hurt her in the least." I paused. "Your daughter is a free spirit. She's a joy to see every month."

As I walked to the nurses' station, I thought, Humphrey, you're enjoying the moment; tonight at the fence you can reflect on Polly's future.

• • •

"**D**octor Humphrey, you have a new admission," Dee said. "Janice Polk is ten, referred in from Fairfax. She's pale, covered with petechiae, and has a peaked look. She's not febrile. They're down in room six. Oh, here are copies of the Fairfax hospital lab slips and a handwritten note from the pediatrician, Doctor Kent, who saw Janice this morning."

I thanked Dee and looked at the lab data; wow—low RBCs, very low platelet count, and all the circulating leukocytes were reported to be lymphoblasts. In the clinical note, Doctor Kent wrote that he had informed the mother that Janice had leukemia. I almost wondered if there was anything left for me to do.

Janice and her mother were both sitting on the bed. I introduced myself to Janice and then her mother.

"I don't like the diagnosis, Doctor Humphrey," Mrs. Polk said in a firm, steady voice, "but after a week of hell, I'm almost relieved to be here. I've known for over five days that something was very, *very* wrong with Janice."

Almost relieved to be on 2 East—this was a first for me. I'd watched and listened to mothers react to their first day on this leukemia ward, but relieved to be here—I was surprised, even a little astonished. I sat on the edge of the bed and started taking notes.

Mrs. Polk provided a very detailed account of the last week: the initial diagnosis of a low-grade infection by their family physician, Doctor Fillmore, and the first antibiotic treatment; the progression of signs and symptoms and the change to a stronger antibiotic; and finally, today, the referral to Doctor Kent.

As we progressed through the surgical, developmental, family, and other components of a complete initial history, Mrs. Polk seemed to relax. Her shoulders dropped, the frown disappeared, and she adjusted the pillow so she could lean back.

During the physical exam, I explained to Janice in simple terms what I was doing, what I found, and what we were going to do to make her feel better. The explanations were also for Mom. It took about thirty minutes.

At the end, Janice looked up at me and observed, "You sure do talk a lot."

That broke what little tension was left. I chuckled. Mom smiled for the first time and told her daughter, "We have a lot to learn, and we're going to be good listeners."

The bone marrow confirmed the clinical diagnosis of acute lymphocytic leukemia, and there were no major problems with the first course of POMP. As Janice began to feel better, she became more comfortable talking to me, making up long stories and pretend adventures.

In May, POMP was again given without any unusual complications, and the same was true in June. I liked both mom and daughter, and we enjoyed each other's company. On our last day together in June, Janice told an unusually long story, and I couldn't resist saying, "Janice, you sure do talk a lot."

• • •

Dee told me Mrs. Yardley had called. "She and her husband want to return to 2 East this week."

"It's Monday. I can get Todd's medical record this morning and reread the autopsy report this afternoon. Anytime Tuesday, Wednesday, or Thursday afternoon would be fine. Please let me know when they'll be here so I can stay on the floor," I said.

"Generally it's only the mothers who return, and only some return," Dee said. She didn't keep track of how many, but she thought most only came back once.

Reading Todd's autopsy report that afternoon, I again noted that the central-nervous-system hemorrhage was assumed to be traumatic but no large leukemic infiltrates or masses were found in the brain. Important, because of Freireich's hope that the high dose of prednisolone in POMP might be effective in inhibiting meningeal leukemia.

Midafternoon on Wednesday, Dee brought Mr. and Mrs. Yardley to the doctors' office. Mrs. Yardley introduced me to Todd's father and stated they didn't want to take up a lot of my time.

I told them I had plenty of time; my chores were done. "I think I've got all the necessary puzzles put together."

We shook hands, and Mr. Yardley reminded me of our earlier telephone conversation. "This is a real journey for me, to see this place that has been so important to my wife and to Todd." He paused. "Important to the whole family," he added.

"And Ralph is also part of the family," I said. Mrs. Yardley brought me up to date on Ralph, her constant companion. I told Mr. Yardley I remembered the second call he had made about the autopsy and that we had learned something important. I explained about leukemic masses in the brains of children. The high doses of the steroid prednisolone might inhibit the formation of such masses. "No masses were found in Todd's brain," I said.

"It's been a real journey for me, too, Doctor Humphrey," Mrs. Yardley said. "I wanted Todd's dad to see this place that I have told him about so often. The respect I have for you and all the nurses. The deep friendships I now have with other mothers. Where so many things happened."

I walked with them to the front doors, shook hands with Mr. Yardley, and told them to please come back anytime.

Opening the door to the floor, I saw Brigid with a child pushing his IV pole. Dee was retying a bathrobe on a little girl. Jerry was sitting on the floor playing some sort of patty-cake game with a three-year-old.

While 2 East might be a place of death, it was also a place of bonding.

• • •

"**G**ood morning, Doctor Humphrey. How are you?" Billy Sullivan asked, extending his right hand.

"Good morning, Billy. I'm fine, and how are you?"

Mrs. Sullivan and I exchanged a smile. Billy wanted to be a grown up.

The interim history and physical exam were unremarkable. Then came the bone marrow and IV. When Billy was ready to be taken back to his room, he was still shedding tears as he sat on the edge of the large surgical table. I asked Billy if he wanted me to carry him. He shook his head. I guessed he thought that was for younger kids, so I lifted him off the table and onto the floor. Asking if I could help with his IV pole, he nodded, and the two of us left the treatment room together, walking side by side down the hall toward his room. Halfway down the hall, Billy reached up and took my hand. My little patient sought comfort from his physical pain.

This simple act transported me back to 1951, working at a summer camp in Wisconsin. There were two college students supervising each cabin of campers, and one developed pneumonia. To help out, I was elevated overnight from stableboy to counselor for ten toilet-trained toddlers.

On a morning when the other counselor had his day off, I had to figure out what to do during the morning free period. Under a willow tree in a light breeze, I told them tales of my childhood and carved each a whistle. As we walked to lunch, the youngest, quietest, and saddest took my hand. My little camper sought comfort from his loneliness.

The significance of these bonding experiences was not lost on me as a stableboy temporarily promoted to cabin counselor or as an internist working on a pediatric floor. Now, decades later, the memory of those little warm hands in mine can still bring a tear to my eyes.

• • •

"Where are the pictures of Erik?" Jerry asked Rick.

"Well, I've had this one on my desk of Erik and Jody since I returned to the floor after my leave for Erik's birth," Rick said, holding up a framed photo.

"What kind of father are you?" Jerry said. "We want to see 'em all!"

Then Jerry and I alternated listing typical first-child shots: Erik in the bathtub, Erik wearing an infant University of Washington T-shirt, Erick in his father's arms, the grandchild in his grandma's arms, Erik with pabulum all over his face, and so on. We then broke into a silly chant: "We want pictures. We want pictures. We want pictures—"

"OK, OK," Rick said, holding his arms up in the surrender pose. With a broad grin on his face, he said he'd bring some in after lunch. "You're going to be sorry."

After Rick left, Jerry said smugly, "I think we just made his day."

Rick returned in two hours with some forty pictures. Rick tried not to belabor each photo, but we wanted the details. He had our undivided attention.

When Rick put the collection back in an envelope, my envy surfaced when I commented that it must be great to be a parent. Jerry concurred.

"What's with the two of you?" Rick asked. "How did you get this far without falling in love and getting married? Do you realize your lives are almost half over?"

Jerry shrugged.

I shook my head.

When Rick said he was sorry and that was none of his business, I told him it was a good question. "My dating started in eighth grade and continued in high school and college, but I never went steady or gave my fraternity pin away. I've never been engaged."

Jerry asked if I ever thought I was in love.

"That started in grad school." I told them about three relationships that I still cherished. "To be honest, at times I do feel lonely, especially after a smooth day here on 2 East, and I've enjoyed watching a mother loving her child, or my getting a hug from a little girl, or watching a toddler smile as I walk into their room—sometimes on these days I ask, 'What if…?'"

"You were in love and never married?" Rick asked, shaking his head.

"Well, there were a number of factors. One was finances, a minor problem; then there was me: I was a workaholic and a planner. I wanted a PhD to give me an extra advantage in an academic career in medicine. But the combined-degree program required long hours, and my dyslexia demanded even more. Yes, I dated, preferred the company of the opposite sex, but these emotional relationships had to fit into my intellectual pursuits."

Jerry started to chuckle and interrupted. "Women don't like to play second fiddle to the structure of DNA."

I nodded and, as an aside, said, "How well I know," and then sighed. "But there's more to it than that," I said. "There was also a strong parental influence. I thought, don't get married until you finish your education, because that's what my parents had done. I saw my parents investing energy in my sister and me. My father didn't spend the weekends playing golf, and my mother wasn't flitting around a pseudo-artistic studio pretending she was creative." I paused and swallowed. "There's a selfish component. When I do take time off, I want to escape. I want to be outdoors: ride a horse, run a river, climb a mountain, ski down a slope, go for a walk, or even talk to a squirrel. These things allow me to be alone."

Jerry's perspective was different. "My parents are my role models for a loving and lasting marriage. At the present time, my emotions are totally consumed by 2 East and seeing young children die of cancer. My heart goes out to each patient, whether the mothers I've caught crying in distant corners of the hospital or the stoic ones who keep it all inside. When I date, I'm self-absorbed. I want to talk about 2 East. I try to project an impersonal perspective and show interest in my partner. But it doesn't take long before I'm babbling on about sick children, getting it off my chest but being a total bore to my date," he said. "I've never had to deal with such emotions before."

Rick didn't interrupt. I was absorbed by Jerry's honesty.

"I want a marriage like my parents' marriage. I consume all of my emotional energy in my own life. I'm not in a situation where I can be a serious partner to anyone else. These days, I date, I party, I drink. I drink too much. But I'm not dating to find a lifelong partner. The women who are willing to put up with my sop are not the kind of people I hope to partner with for the long term. Next year, we'll leave 2 East and move on to our laboratory projects. I anticipate that I'll return to being a person who can separate his day job from his personal life. I look forward to being able to leave my burdens at the office and share meaningful time with a life partner. In short, I didn't plan it this way, but I've put my personal life on hold."

"I suppose I shouldn't be surprised that the two of you aren't married. Most of the guys from my residency and fellowship weren't married," Rick said. Then, abandoning his usual decorum, he added, "I don't remember any of them training a horse, but they did chase after women."

That ended our discussions about marriage.

• • •

The conversation about marriage haunted me as I approached the fence. Rick was married; in his private life he was investing his energy in his family. "Easy to accept," I said to Domino.

You don't do that, Humphrey. Is it because you can't? You don't know how? Is it because of your training or your role models in medicine? Some sort of coping strategy? More frightening was the possibility that these emotions were just not there.

A simile from my reading of Eastern philosophy rose from my subconscious. Did I exist as a lump of clay that had no purpose until I was thrown as a bowl, and it was the emptiness in the middle that gave usefulness to who I was?

I started to chuckle. You're tired and being foolish or sentimental. The chuckle turned to light laughter. Here you are talking to a horse, and that's better than fabricating feelings for a psychiatrist or blowing your brains out.

"I always enjoy these little chats, Domino. You stay out here and enjoy the pasture, and I'll go inside and go to bed…'perchance to dream'…"

MAY

Two more months. Following the POMP protocol, I'd stopped treatment on two children who might well be cured of what was formerly a fatal cancer. Are you ever going to do anything that important in the future? Time for you, Humphrey, to stop being holier-than-thou about laboratory research.

• • •

Clinical research on controlling infections in children with low white counts was a high priority for Jay, and he pursued the problem.

Jerry presented a four-year-old girl, Susan, with granulocytopenia, fever, and a positive blood culture for a bacterium called *Klebsiella*. Jerry hoped the marrow would recover and start producing granulocytes.

"There may be something else we can do while we're waiting for her marrow to recover," Jay said. "We've learned that the granulocytes from patients with philadelphia chromosome-positive chronic granulocytic leukemia or CGL can ingest and kill bacteria just like normal granulocytes." Jay explained that during the chronic phase of CGL when the white count was anywhere from fifty thousand to a million cells, these patients could donate blood for patients with sepsis. "What's your patient's blood type?"

Jerry flipped through the chart. "Susan's A positive."

Breaking Little Bones

Looking at small notebook he carried, Jay smiled. "We're following a fifty-year-old patient named Charles Russell: he has CGL, he is philadelphia chromosome-positive, he's A positive, his last WBC was one hundred twenty-five thousand, and he's willing to donate blood." Jay was excited. "Call the blood bank and ask for a cross match between your little girl and Mr. Russell, and we'll work out a way to harvest just the white blood cells to keep the volume of the transfusion appropriate for a child. If there's a match, call me."

After rounds, Rick asked Jerry about the philadelphia chromosome; he knew there had been some excitement about chromosomal abnormality but hadn't read in depth about either CGL or the chromosome findings.

Jerry explained that in the adult literature a lot was written about this abnormality, first described in Philadelphia. The anomaly was a shorter-than-normal twenty-second chromosome, which could be observed with a light microscope. It was specific for CGL and not found in other leukemias.

After finding out that there was a match between Susan and Mr. Russell, Jay laid out a plan: bone marrow before the infusion of Mr. Russell's blood into Susan and then a daily CBC. If there were any signs of granulocyte production, the bone-marrow aspirate was to be repeated. Jay explained that it was important to know if the granulocytes in Susan's blood were from her marrow cells or from grafted CGL cells.

On the second posttransfusion day, there were a few granulocytes, and more the third day. A marrow aspirate on the third day demonstrated the presence of the philadelphia chromosome in some of Susan's bone-marrow cells, and when her marrow recovered a week later, the philadelphia chromosome-positive cells disappeared. There had been a temporary graft. Mr. Russell's CGL cells were growing in Susan's marrow and producing granulocytes to fight the sepsis. When Susan recovered and produced her own granulocytes, she also produced immune competent cells. Mr. Russell's grafted cells were then rejected. Jay had followed this daily, and each day he smiled. Jay generally didn't smile during rounds.

When it was all over, Jerry said, "What an important set of scientific observations!"

Rick chuckled. "Isn't it more important that Susan is afebrile and off antibiotics?"

"Well," Jerry said sarcastically, "what can you expect from a pediatrician?"

• • •

After presenting a six-year-old boy with sepsis and neutropenia on rounds, Rick asked Jay if there was a CML donor whose blood type was B positive. The answer was no. "It's too bad we can't harvest normal granulocytes."

To our amazement, Jay said, "We're working on that right now. Come over to my lab around eleven, and I'll show you a machine that we think will allow the isolation of normal granulocytes for transfusion into granulocytopenic patients in the future."

After Jay left, Rick said, "That's got to be impossible."

"Yeah," I said, "but remember that's what they said about transfusing platelets."

"But, Ben," Jerry interrupted, "look at the number of cells in a cc of blood and couple that with the biological life span of each cell type. We've been transfusing red blood cells for decades. Big deal. There're millions of 'em, and the life span is, shall we say, a hundred days. Now for platelets, we have fewer numbers and a shorter life span. There are a few hundred thousand platelets in a cc, and their life span is something like ten days. OK, so Jay solved that problem, and we've been giving platelets for a few years. But granulocytes! There're only a few thousand in a cc, and the life span is less than ten hours! Do the math, Ben; there just aren't that many granulocytes in a liter of normal blood."

Breaking Little Bones

At a quarter past eleven, Jay took us to a laboratory. Next to one wall, near an electrical outlet, was a white three-cubic-foot machine. There was an instrument panel on the back, with controls for temperature, rotational speed, infusion rates for blood and heparinized saline as well as several controls for harvesting. Above the control panel were two plastic bags, one containing blood and the other saline. Tubing from each bag was connected to the machine. Looking down into the cube, one could see a large spinning disk containing blood. Red blood cells are denser than white blood cells, and these were present as a red ring at the outer edge of the disk. Above the red ring was a tan ring of plasma. In between was a thin cream-colored ring, the so-called buffy coat of white blood cells.

A technician was busy collecting samples from the disk, adjusting various controls and keeping a record of all adjustments. Jay patted the side of the machine as one would thump a bird dog. Standing there on four legs, this was his albino retriever.

After listening to a description of the machine's functions, we went back to Jay's office. He explained that an engineer from IBM had approached him about collecting human white blood cells. The engineer's adolescent son had developed leukemia, and, as a concerned father, he had learned about blood banking and the lack of white-blood-cell transfusions to fight infections.

"I was a little skeptical at first," Jay admitted, "but eventually thought it was worth a try. Right now we're experimenting with expired bank blood, but the long-range plan will be for continuous flow centrifugation. The donor's blood will flow into the machine, the buffy coat harvested, and the plasma and harvested red blood cells returned to the donor as fresh blood keeps flowing out of the donor into the machine. That's why we're calling the process 'continuous flow centrifugation.' The donor will have to stay hooked up to the machine for a couple of hours. Right now we don't know exactly how long."

We were impressed. When we reached 2 East, Jerry said, "I'll be goddamned."

G. Bennett Humphrey

Only Jay would be willing to take on harvesting granulocytes when most hematologists would say, "That's impossible." I reminded myself that a lot of clinicians were saying, "We'll never be able to cure leukemia."

• • •

On the Thursday after the demonstration of the white-blood-cell separator, the sun was setting when I got back to Kirkhill. My mind was still busy with a problem from 2 East. Tomorrow was Friday, discharge day, and Robert 'Gosh' Thurman had a very low white count; I hoped he wouldn't spike a fever. A ride on Domino would be a good distraction, so I hopped on his broad, fat back. My mind wasn't on Domino, and he sensed that. A slight kick of his hindquarters was ignored, and he tossed me over his ears; I landed on the third finger of my left hand.

I knew it was broken. I bent the handle of a large spoon to form a curved splint and taped my finger to the handle and the bowl to my palm. I took two aspirin and went to bed. It served me right: don't ruminate over your problems while riding a horse.

Next morning I went to Bethesda Naval Hospital, where the clinical associates went for health care.

"Well, Commander, it's broken just where you thought it would be," said the naval corpsman. "You can wait around for one of the orthopedic surgeons, or I can fix you up with a finger splint and you can be on your way, sir."

It wasn't every day of the week that I was called Commander. I enjoyed the manner of this enlisted man. "Let me see the x-ray," I said in a pleasant but professional manner. "A simple fracture with minimal displacement," I observed. "Go ahead and put my finger in a splint."

"Yes, sir."

The splint was fashioned to my finger and my hand wrapped in an elastic dressing. "Careful how you use that hand for the next two weeks, sir. Any problems, and we'll be glad to see you again. Anytime of the day or night, sir."

"Well done. Thank you," I said in the best military tone I could muster.

On the way to the door, the corpsman asked, "Are you going to sell that horse, sir?"

"No. He's not difficult—only a bit of a character. I hate to admit it, but that horse is a pony."

I could hold a pen and write notes and orders, but doing a bone-marrow aspiration was not possible. Carl Shively was in clinic, and Rick volunteered to do the procedure for me. I forewarned Rick, "Mrs. Shively is a real character. I never know what she's going to say."

After I held up my left hand with the splinted third finger, I explained that Doctor Lottsfeldt would do the marrow.

"Weeell, Doctor Humphrey," Mrs. Shively said, "did you have that finger someplace it didn't belong?" We both laughed while Rick picked up his jaw from the floor.

Walking down the hall with the marrow specimen, Rick said, "Did you *hear* what she said?"

"Yes," I said. "I've never thought about this before, but she's a real human being. You and I are veneered with etiquette."

• • •

After a midday ride, I was cleaning tack when Frank came out of the cabin to tell me that Jerry was on the phone. That was odd; it was Sunday, and I didn't have a child in the hospital.

Jerry said Joshua Anderson had been admitted for a course of POMP to be started tomorrow. That part wasn't unusual, but Joshua's mom had told one of the other mothers she was carrying a gun. "I don't know this woman, Ben. Will you come in and talk to her?"

"I'll be right there."

After cleaning up, I asked Frank if he would put away the tack, and I jumped into the Healey. As I drove, I had a chance to think about Mrs. Anderson. Joshua had been diagnosed in January. I couldn't think of any remark by Mrs. Anderson suggesting that she was angry with me. Like Joshua, she always addressed me as sir and often said that the nurses and the doctors on 2 East were in her prayers. By the time I arrived, I remembered that Joshua's dad was a sheriff and Joshua played with toy guns. I also had a plan—a dumb plan.

Barbara was in the nurses' station. I explained why I had come in and asked Barbara to call security and request that an officer be on standby.

Then, like a damn fool, I knocked on the door and walked into Joshua's room. I found myself looking down the barrel of a six-shooter. I put my hands up, and Joshua dropped his toy gun on the bed. That was our routine. After saying hello to Mrs. Anderson, she closed her Bible and gave me her undivided attention—another routine. I told Joshua this was just a social call and his mother and I needed to do some paperwork.

Mrs. Anderson listened to my comment that carrying a pistol or a revolver was against the rules of the hospital. Her response was, "Last time we was here, a nigger got real smart with me. I told my husband, and he give me this twenty-five automatic to carry. This is a big city, you know. Nobody bothers me in our small town."

I tried not to wince. I knew the word of course but had never before heard it used as if there were no other way to refer to a black person. When asked, she said that she felt safe here in the hospital, and Mrs. Anderson agreed to let security keep the revolver until Joshua was discharged.

I found Jerry in the doctors' office and told him what had happened. I realized I needed to unwind before I drove home. I had a tight feeling in my gut. I grabbed a bag of peanuts and went to see Son of Squirrel.

He scampered down his tree, took a peanut, and ran a safe distance away to eat his prize.

Why had I come in? Jerry could have called security. I certainly didn't come in to prove I was brave. Asking Mrs. Anderson to surrender a weapon was a bit foolish. Finally the answer came to me; I came in because Jerry asked me to.

• • •

Being on 2 East was teaching me a lot about medicine, research, and myself, but today, I was reminded of where I was living. Mrs. Anderson used the N-word as a matter of course. That night at the fence, I thought about history and the segregation—no, not segregation—the whole racial-hatred problem.

When I was a preschooler, my mother made it clear there were some totally unacceptable words for *Negro*, and those terms, like dirty words and swearwords, would not be tolerated. My grade school was WASP white, but approximately one-quarter of the high-school population was black. On the athletic field and in the band and orchestra, only talent counted. I didn't make a single black acquaintance during high school.

There were black undergraduate students at the University of Illinois but not many. I remembered an incident when a barber refused to cut a black student's hair.

During my graduate-school years at the University of Chicago, I did have black friends and went on a few dates with a black undergraduate from Alabama who worked one summer in Goldwasser's laboratory.

What came to me this night at the fence were the ugly stories in the northern newspapers. One was about Emmett Till in the 1950s and more recently James Chaney and two white civil-rights workers in Mississippi. But I thought of these as problems of the Deep South.

While I thought of Vietnam as a parallel to the war against leukemia, there was yet another war was playing out. Americans were marching in Selma, Alabama, and to the Washington Mall.

• • •

B rigid handed me a chart and a thin medical record. "We admitted Michelle Karr this morning at seven forty-five."
"It's Wednesday!"
Brigid's eyes were full of unfallen tears. I was tempted to touch her forearm but nodded instead. Despite having dated Brigid, I was trained not to do that, so I said, "Thank you." I had to swallow hard after saying it.

In Michelle's room, Dee was sitting next to Mrs. Karr, holding her hand, and Michelle was on her mother's lap. I didn't say anything. Mrs. Karr opened Michelle's gown. Petechiae everywhere.

At the sink, I washed my hands, wondering, God, what am I going to say? Michelle was not febrile to my touch, her spleen was enlarged, and so was her liver. "I'll do a marrow right away."

"Is that really necessary?" Mrs. Karr asked, knowing that her daughter had relapsed.

I told Mrs. Karr a relapse was defined by a bone-marrow aspiration and we didn't want to make an assumption. Mrs. Karr said she understood.

At 9:20 a.m., John Thomas called me from the path lab. "Ben, the marrow on Michelle Karr is a full-blown relapse. I don't see any normal cells—only lymphoblasts."

"Ben?" John asked.

"I'm still on the line."

"Do you want to come up?"

My initial reaction was no, and then the reality struck. All the mothers knew I looked at my marrows, and it would be better for me to tell

Mrs. Karr that the pathologist and I agreed. I again thought, what will I say now that Michelle has relapsed?

At 9:50 a.m., Mrs. Karr told me she and her husband had already talked about further therapy; they didn't want Michelle to receive daunomycin. They had also talked to their pediatrician, who was very willing to help with terminal care so that Michelle and her mother could be home, close to friends and family. There was no long discussion; IV therapy had been hell for Michelle; infants have very few veins near the surface of the skin. Wednesday's child went home, and that evening I went to the fence. If my reaction was a feeling of emptiness, I could only wonder what kind of hell Mrs. Karr was going through.

• • •

Ah, Hilary's name was on the Board, which meant a chance to catch up on what her brothers were doing. Hilary, Liam, and Brendan were a triple treat.

I said hello to Hilary, was rewarded with a smile, and then turned to greet her brothers, but before I could say anything, Brendon stepped forward to show me that his right arm was in a cast. He was obviously proud of this white badge of courage and handed me a marking pen.

"Do you want me to sign your cast?"

Brendon frowned, and his mother explained that I meant his "plaster."

To contribute to this confusion of the English language, I asked Brendon if he had been run over by a lorry.

"Oh no!" Brendon exclaimed. "I fell down while Liam was chasing me."

Smiling, I said I knew he hadn't been run over by a lorry. I explained that when I was traveling in England and Ireland, I learned new European-English words for common American-English words. "Now, Brendon, you've taught me another: *plaster* for *cast*."

I told Liam his eye looked as good as new. He just frowned. Another attempt to engage him in a conversation didn't work. I asked Mrs. O'Keefe what was wrong.

"Hilary has you as her special doctor, and Brendon now has an orthopedic surgeon, but Liam doesn't have a doctor."

I couldn't think of anything to say; this was not something to joke about.

During my lunch break, I told Son of Squirrel, "You know, sometimes it's better to have pain than to be left out."

• • •

"We've got to go for coffee," Jerry said. He was like a kid with a secret. "Are you dating anyone?"

"No."

"Then I've found the perfect girl for you. Her name's Sandy. Listen to this: undergraduate BA from University of Virginia, a year studying in France, currently working on a master's degree in foreign relations at Georgetown University and learning Arabic. In high school she had her own horse; she's five eight, and she's striking, not flashy, a quiet, sophisticated beauty with a sense of humor, charming…"

Holding up a hand, I said, "Whoa! Something's gotta be wrong. Is it body odor, bad teeth, shaving a mustache off her upper lip every morning—"

"No, no, no," Jerry said. "Sandy isn't going out much because of her studies. But when I mentioned your graduate work, your postdoc in Germany, your Thoroughbred, and that you're a romantic, Sandy said she'd like to meet you. Here's her number."

We met in her small Georgetown apartment; she was everything Jerry had described. If she was wearing makeup, it wasn't apparent. Jerry had forgotten to mention her long face with classical features, hazel-brown eyes, and pleasing figure.

While Sandy collected her purse, I admired her apartment's décor and was especially struck by a work area on the far wall opposite a bank of windows that looked out on a tree-lined street. An eight-foot-long flat surface was supported by two drawer filing cabinets, with an electric typewriter in the center and, at each end of the table, swivel fluorescent lamps.

"I try to spend four hours here each morning. This is the center of my universe, and my peripheral vision is limited to those filing cabinets. Most of my guests don't even notice this area, but Jerry told me you have a PhD, so you must've also written a dissertation."

"Yes, it's quite an experience."

When we got to the Healey, I opened the door for her, and she asked, "Can we put the top down?" When I agreed, she suggested, "If you go to the other side, I'll help you with the top." Then with a coquettish smile, she said, "I'm perfectly capable of hopping into the front seat and can even close the door myself."

I laughed. "OK. But I would prefer to open the car door for you when we get to the restaurant."

She winked and said, "Deal!"

During dinner we exchanged our plans for the future. "I have to finish my master's degree, take and pass the foreign-service exam, and then work in some North African country for at least two or three years." She shook her head. "And you?"

"Next year I'll be in a laboratory, then I need to finish my third year of residency in internal medicine, and thereafter—a two-year fellowship in hematology." I chuckled. "Then, I can look for a job."

The rest of the evening flowed effortlessly. We were no longer on our first date. The dating personae were set aside. We each had funny stories to tell about living in Europe and learning to speak a foreign language. We had spent an hour on a date and for the next two hours just enjoyed each other's company, but there would be no second date, no future for us. We would part as we had met: two loners with unfinished business, busy with our careers, and not wanting a marital entanglement. Sandy wasn't perfect; she was just like me.

• • •

Tuesday rounds with Freireich ran smoothly until Jerry said his two children were on schedule but that a seven-year-old named Thomas Loken was extremely hypoplastic, no leukemic cells but no normal cells.

With a steady gaze, Jay looked at Jerry as if to say, "Haven't we been through this before?" but he said nothing.

That ended rounds, and after Jay left, Jerry was obviously upset. He wanted to go for coffee. He needed to get off of 2 East.

"I'm going to spend the rest of my academic life dealing with medical students, residents, and fellows in hematology-oncology, and all I've learned from Freireich is how not to be abrasive," Jerry said, hitting the table with a closed fist.

I lowered my head, sighed, and then said, "I enjoy teaching. It's one reason I want to go into academic medicine."

"I'm still smarting from my wish to stop methotrexate on Jennifer Johnson," Rick said. "Remember, I told him I was trained to stop therapy, and he told me I wasn't in Minnesota. I'm a pediatrician, and I've had two good years of training in pediatric oncology. Jay's an internist. He's got one approach to the development of therapy: damn the toxicity, maximum doses of four drugs, hope for a leap forward for a cure."

"Well said, Rick," Jerry inserted. "You're right."

"Yeah, but the focus should be on the children of 2 East, not on whether Jay's got an abrasive personality," I said. "OK, Jay's got one approach. What's an alternative way of developing therapy?"

"The cooperative groups have been evaluating two-drug combinations," Rick said. "Why not start using three-drug combos? You're trained in research, Ben. What do you think?"

"Rick, I'd like to think I've been exposed to very good laboratory research with molecules and cell biology in animals. My PhD advisor, Gene Goldwasser, was excellent, and he was a hell of a nice guy. But during med school and my residency, I was not exposed to any clinical research. Now on 2 East, I've been given a big dose of it. They're two very different worlds."

"What've you gotten out of the year so far, Ben?" Jerry asked with a sigh.

"I've learned something painful and positive from Jay," I said. "He got it right: control of bleeding—hemorrhagic deaths had to be solved first before developing curative chemotherapy. We know Jay did a lot of research on platelets, and when he gave platelet concentrates to the first three patients, they all died. The autopsy reports didn't implicate platelet infusions as the cause of death, so Jay had the guts to give the fourth and fifth platelet infusion. I wouldn't have had the balls to do that."

Rick cleared his throat. "OK, Ben, but controlling bleeding doesn't justify developing toxic—or more important, *fatal* chemotherapy. Our first month here on 2 East, I watched a beautiful little girl slowly die of a progressive staph infection. I know I've told you this before. I don't want to ever again see another Jennifer Johnson."

"Neither do I," Jerry said.

After I echoed the statement, Jerry said to me, "Ben, if you had been in charge of research developing platelet infusions, you could have given the fourth and fifth platelet infusions without being an abrasive son of a bitch."

"I once asked Dee about the days before platelet transfusion," I said. "She said she almost quit. 'We changed the blood-soaked sheets and pillowcases in the morning and went home at night with bloodstained uniforms.' I of course had never witnessed that, but in April, I told Mrs. Sullivan and both Mr. and Mrs. Thompkins that we were stopping therapy on Sally and Sarah. Both moms wanted therapy stopped because they'd seen the toxicity of POMP. Mr. Thompkins, who had never spent any time on 2 East, wanted therapy continued, but Sarah's mother prevailed. She mentioned Jennifer Johnson. Both girls are now in follow-up to see if they're cured."

"You're saying we need to wait until the results are in on POMP before we judge Freireich?" was Rick's response. "That's something I couldn't have considered last fall, Ben."

The conversation had become heavy, and we were in need of some humor, so I said, "You've been very diplomatic in this exchange. You haven't said it, so I'll say it for you. 'I'm just another one of those goddamn fucking internists.'"

Jerry laughed.

Rick smiled and put his hands up in a semisurrender position.

We got up, returned our empty coffee cups to the dirty-dish tray, and went back to 2 East, our children, and our clinical research responsibilities.

• • •

"This is a typical presentation of Burkitt's or African Lymphoma," Doctor Bell said as a colored slide flashed on the screen. My stomach was suddenly queasy as I stared in disbelief at the grossly distorted face of a young African child.

The right side of the face was swollen—no, more like the skin was stretched over a large tumor mass. The right eye was displaced anteriorly, the lids were swollen, and an exudate ran down the cheek; the conjunctiva and iris could not be seen due to an irregular red mass that protruded between the lids. The tumor extended down to the lower jaw, distorting the lips. I found it hard to listen to the speaker as he commented that the tumor could invade the abdomen and central nervous system.

"This pediatric tumor was first described in 1958 by Denis Burkitt, a surgeon working in Uganda. It was thought to be an undifferentiated sarcoma but was later established as a lymphoma." He discussed a series of pathology slides.

"The tumor is endemic to equatorial Africa. Of special interest is the association of the tumor with *falciparum* malaria," Doctor Bell said. "This tumor is not found at higher elevations or in very dry regions where mosquitoes are not found."

The next quarter of an hour was spent discussing the possible viral etiology of this lymphoma. "Last year in March, viral particles were reported in a Burkitt's lymphoma cell line by an expert electron microscopist, Doctor Epstein." Doctor Bell explained that his laboratory in the Division of Molecular Biology wanted to examine fresh tissue from a patient and arrangements had been made with authorities in Nigeria for a patient to be flown to Washington. "The patient will be admitted to 2 East. After an excisional biopsy has been obtained, the patient will be transferred to the Cancer Chemotherapy Service for a trial of therapy. Doctor Freireich has been reviewing the few case reports of patients receiving anticancer drugs." Doctor Bell fumbled through his notes. "I'm told there is tumor reduction with a drug…called methotrexate."

The three of us rode down in the elevator to 2 East.

"Do you think Bell knows anything about children?" Rick asked.

"It's not a child, Rick; it's a patient transporting fresh tumor tissue," I said.

As we walked on to 2 East, Dee came down the hall to meet us. "Doctor Sandler, Doctor Freireich wants you to care for a child from Nigeria. She's seven and will arrive next Tuesday."

"I think I'll start reading about Nigeria," Jerry said.

• • •

At half past eight Tuesday morning, Jerry asked, "Ben, will you cover for me?" He explained that the Nigerian embassy was sending a car to the Clinical Center. "A member of its staff, a Mr. Salawu, is taking me to Dulles International Airport to meet the patient. He seems like a nice guy and speaks her language, Ibo. He'll even spend some time up here on 2 East."

During the previous week, Jerry had been doing his homework. Rick and I enjoyed listening to Jerry tell us about the country, its languages, cultures, and history.

At half past eleven, Jerry walked into the office, dropped a chart on his desk, and sat down with a thud. He buried his face into his hands and then swept them over his scalp.

"Let me tell you about this little girl," Jerry said. "The left side of her face is as distorted as the picture we saw last week—no, more so. The tumor is in the upper jaw; it displaces the nose; the eye on that side is swollen shut; her upper-central incisors protrude through her mouth, and the teeth are spread apart by the tumor. She can close her mouth and drink fluids."

Rick and I just looked at each other.

Jerry took a deep breath and continued. "That's not the worst part! She's trembling all over, she looks with her one open eye from one individual to another, and now that's she's here on the floor, she no longer responds to Mr. Salawu." Jerry explained that arrangements had been made for both parents to accompany their daughter to NIH, but when they got to the airport, the mother refused to get out of the car. Apparently it was quite a scene, and they decided to send the child on alone so something could be done about her tumor.

"Mr. Salawu's in there right now, and Dee is working out a plan with the nurses on how to gain the child's confidence and get her to relax a bit."

Mr. Salawu taught Dee and Brigid to say *good* and the equivalent of *OK* in Ibo. Because her first name was difficult to pronounce, rather than everyone on the floor mispronouncing it, Mr. Salawu explained to the girl that everyone would call her Alice.

"We're going to feed her first," Dee said. "Then we'll see if she likes having her feet washed, and thereafter hopefully we'll give her a full bath."

"That's great," Jerry said. "Why don't you spend a couple of hours working with Alice? Let me know if I can help. I'll do a simple exam on her this afternoon."

After Dee left, Rick said, "Can you imagine what that child is going through?"

"No," Jerry said in a deep voice. "Mr. Salawu's doing his best. On the way to the airport, he taught me a few phrases and gave me this Ibo-English language guide."

We were all down in the dumps, so I asked to see the Ibo phrase book, opened it, and pretended to read. "Here's something useful: 'Have you seen any rhinos running around here lately?'"

• • •

In the early afternoon, the three of us were standing outside Alice's room.

According to Jerry, the nurses had performed a miracle: she no longer trembled, and her lips could form a smile on the right on her face. Her stare was no longer wide-eyed but a steady gaze. "When I said hello in Ibo and extended my hand, she lightly grasped a few fingers and nodded. You guys need to meet her—one at a time."

After we practiced saying hello in Ibo, Rick and I each took a turn. Rick went in first and came out in a few minutes shaking his head as if in wonder.

"She was dehydrated," Jerry observed. "Lunch has probably started to correct that. We can use her urine-specific gravity to monitor her state of rehydration. I want to avoid any needles today. I'm going to talk to Jay about that right now."

Before we split up, Jamie, a dietician, stopped us in the hall. "What a challenge! She's the most rewarding patient I ever helped with a meal," Jamie said, almost crying.

Alice had eaten very little from the standard lunch tray, but she did manage a square of Jell-O. When the dieticians heard about this, they put together a tray of Jell-O, pudding, tapioca, and yogurt.

"She ate all of what we brought up," Jamie said and smiled. "Poor thing. She must not have eaten anything on the plane. I have the feeling she likes yellow food. Almost as if yellow is more important than taste. I have an idea—"

"Who's writing orders on my patient?" It was Doctor Bell. All four of us turned and looked down at him. Bell was short of stature, among other things.

After Jerry said he was responsible for orders, Bell continued, "Doctor, I need blood drawn right now for these tests and blood drawn tomorrow morning." He handed Jerry two slips of paper.

Bell interrupted Jerry's attempt to read through the lists. "Doctor, those are all tests I need for my virology studies. You don't need to know why they are ordered; just draw the blood."

With that, Rick folded his arm across his chest. Mount Rainier was not happy. "Doctor Bell. That's Doctor Sandler. He's planning on seeing Doctor Freireich this afternoon about this child's schedule," Rick said slowly and distinctly.

I'd never seen Rick like this before.

"Doctor. I don't have time to make an appointment to see Jay Freireich," Bell said. "The cost of keeping a patient on this floor is high, and it's coming out of my budget. I've asked the surgeons to put her on the schedule for tomorrow morning."

The top came off of Mount Rainier. Rick stepped forward. "We don't *need* an appointment to see Doctor Freireich. When it comes to taking care of the *children* on this floor, his door is always open. We value his advice, Doctor Bell."

Jerry diplomatically suggested they go to Jay's office. Jerry asked me to call Jay and tell him that he and Doctor Bell were on the way.

On the phone in the nurses' station, I told Jay what was up, and he said he'd take care of the problem.

Twenty minutes later, Jerry walked into the office chuckling and wiping tears from his eyes. "God, I love Emil J. Freireich, MD," Jerry cried. "Jay was brilliant! He greeted Bell as if he were glad to see him. Told Bell he knew how important all this was and that he didn't want anything to go wrong. Jay told Bell, 'In fact, I'll go over to 2 East right now, and we'll work out a schedule.' It didn't take him two minutes to get Bell off 2 East."

Rick and I listened with delight.

"What got into you, Rick?" Jerry asked. "You never lose your cool."

"Meeting Alice got to me," Rick said. "She needs the best care we can give her. Not the fastest handling we think we can get away with."

"The same thing happened to Jay," Jerry said. "When she smiled and touched his fingers—well—I've never seen Jay smile like that. When I left the room, Jay told me, 'You're right. No needles today, no surgery tomorrow.'"

The three of us were enjoying the moment when a clinical associate from surgery stormed in the office. "What the hell is the meaning of this 'emergency—high priority' excisional biopsy?" he demanded. "We've got a full schedule tomorrow! Is Bell an MD or a PhD?"

Jerry calmed him down. He told the young surgeon that Bell was a virologist and then shared some of the more humorous events of the afternoon.

"These damn PhDs," the surgeon said with a smile. "'Piled higher and deeper,' as we say."

Half a smile and a gentle touching of fingers had won the day.

• • •

Alice became a "Child of the Floor." As with Jeff Donaldson and Betty Miller, a few of the mothers did their best to support Alice. Someone had the bright idea of teaching her to put together simple puzzles. Apparently, she had never seen a puzzle before and at first liked to watch the picture being assembled.

With a little coaching, Alice could put together a six-piece puzzle. After Dee told me about this, she smiled and said, "You know, one of these moms is very southern. I think Alice has torn down a racial barrier."

"This is the first Negro child we've had on the floor," I said and frowned.

"There have been others. NIH has absolutely no racial barriers," Dee said. "Doctor Karon has said he thinks the small number is a function of Negroes not having access to health care."

The attention of the other mothers started the morning of Alice's second day. That same afternoon, Rick and I were in the hall listening to drum music coming out of her room. Standing outside Alice's door was Edward, one of Rick's three-year-old patients. He had one hand on his IV pole and the other taped to an IV board held parallel to the floor. Edward couldn't do much with his hands, but he could bounce his bottom from side to side in time with the rhythm.

Noting our delight, Morgan told us, "Doctor S. found a record of Nigerian drum music, and the audiovisual people brought down a record player. Edward's not the only one who's got rhythm. The whole floor's jumping."

Back in the doctors' office, Rick congratulated Jerry, who said that a girl he was dating played the guitar and tonight she'd play for Alice.

Later, Dee found one more way to brighten Alice's day. In the girl's suitcase, Dee found a long bright-blue dress and matching hat and showed them to Alice, who smiled and pointed to the outfit with a little jump. The nurses helped Alice get into her dress and hat. Rick and I each went in to admire the outfit, touch the fabric, and smile in approval. Jerry got out his Nigerian phrase book and looked up *beautiful*.

Jerry worked very hard to learn some Ibo. That second day, when Mr. Salawu from the embassy came by, he told Jerry that Alice had said she thought she was learning some English because she could almost understand what Jerry was saying. Rick and I laughed. Jerry had a marvelous way of being able to laugh at himself.

Jerry's smile turned to a pensive frown, and he said, "Yeah, tomorrow Alice is going for that biopsy."

• • •

Alice returned from surgery with her head wrapped in an elastic bandage. There was a bulge over what we assumed was the biopsy site. She didn't respond to the nurses, or to the mothers who tried to entertain her with a puzzle, or to drum music. Most distressing was her not wanting to eat.

On the second postoperative day, one of the surgical associates and Jerry removed the dressing, inspected the sutures in the excision site, measured the tumor mass, and applied a fresh dressing. The concern was not only infection but also tumor growth, which could cause the sutures to be pulled loose and the surgical incision to open, a wound dehiscence. POMP therapy might cause tumor shrinkage, but would chemotherapy interfere with wound healing?

On the third day post-op, Jerry's measurements indicated the tumor was growing. A senior surgeon came down to see Alice, and he, Jay, and Jerry conferred at the bedside. There was no experience to draw on. POMP was started that afternoon.

On the second day of POMP, Dee burst into the office without knocking. "Doctor Sandler!"

Jerry was out the door. Twenty minutes later he returned. "Alice vomited up some roundworms. They're not only in the vomit but also coming out her nose. When I got to her room, she was screaming, crying, and trembling worse than when she was admitted."

Rick and I didn't say anything.

"We cleaned Alice up, and I gave her a sedative. POMP must be toxic to the worms; I just hope this doesn't continue all day."

Later Jerry told us the migration of the worms seemed to be over, and Alice was sleeping.

311

She had not eaten since surgery; now she was vomiting and losing weight. On the fourth day of POMP, the wound dehisced. Now the surgeons came every day to pack the open wound.

Everybody hoped that, with the completion of POMP therapy, Alice would start to eat, but she didn't. POMP didn't cause dramatic tumor reduction. We knew that Jerry was despondent as he was first on the floor in the morning, in and out of Alice's room, and the last to leave in the evening. About the only thing he'd volunteered was, "She's lost weight again today."

Five days after the completion of POMP, Jay and Jerry decided not to give Alice another course. Arrangements were made to fly Alice back to Nigeria. One of the women from the embassy, a nurse, would accompany Alice on the flight home.

Jerry and Dee accompanied Alice as she was wheeled off of the floor. The walls of 2 East were dark. I don't think I've ever seen the hall that dark.

• • •

After Alice left the floor, Jerry wanted to talk about her. We all wanted to talk about Alice.

Rick said, "I lost my cool in my defense of Alice. I'm glad that's still possible."

"I've been dating a wonderful gal, Judy, who plays the guitar and has a beautiful voice," Jerry said. "I told her about Alice. The night before surgery, she came up to 2 East and sang to her. It was clear that Alice was taken with the music, and so was I. Afterward, we went to a small restaurant. Just before we were served, Judy started to cry, not just tears but sobbing, and she said, 'Alice is going to die.'"

I closed a journal I had been reading, and Rick set a chart aside.

"When I told Judy we were doing research to try to cure these children, she told me, 'But right now, they're all going to die.' We're hardened professionals, and it took Judy, this wonderful human being, to point out what 2 East is all about."

"*Hardened.* That's more provocative than *being trained to be professional,*" Rick said.

"I've never used that word before," I said. "I've thought of myself as trying to be objective, but *hardened* might be the right word. The way to get through the day: bone-marrow aspirates, writing POMP orders, looking for toxicity, telling a parent there's been a relapse, and then in the next room saying, 'Everything's all right, and you're going home today.'"

"Yeah," Jerry said. "Diagnosis, prognosis, notes in the clinical charts: the mechanics of treatment. But in between, there's time for caring, empathy, and worrying. Then in the evening I escape, barhopping, dating, dining out."

During the day, I couldn't reflect on 2 East. It took time for me to wind down. It was in the evening with the horses, when I was alone, that I tried to make sense of my day.

"If I've had a really bad day," Rick said, "I'll go home and get Erik out of his crib. Even if he's asleep, I'll sit down and just hold him."

• • •

The responses of children returning to 2 East varied. Some of the young ones cried or screamed or were carried sobbing onto the floor. A few would run to the nurses' station to ask if a friend was on the floor. Some of the older children vented anger or responded by withdrawing for a few hours.

Almost all the mothers formed friendships with others. Most of the kids developed tight friendships, but there was a difference. The mothers used the telephone, so they knew who was doing well and who had relapsed or died.

On a Thursday morning, Rick said, "Hey, you two, I've got something I should share." This wasn't like Rick. He explained that a six-year-old named Sam was admitted on Sunday night. His parents always brought him in on Sunday so that POMP could be started early Monday, facilitating an early discharge Friday. Jerry asked if Sam was the little guy that generally had a toy train in his hand, and Rick nodded.

"Cute kid," Jerry said.

"This week, the nurses knew that the floor was going to be full on Monday; a couple of kids would have to be transferred to 12 East. So they scheduled Sam to go because he tolerated POMP and was an easygoing kid, and as one of the nurses said, 'Sam always fits in with whatever's going on.'"

"When Sam was told he'd be up on 12 East, he screamed, fell to the floor, and pounded it with his fists and feet. They couldn't calm him down and immediately told him they'd send someone else. The panic abated, but the terror continued. He didn't want the nurses near him, especially Barbara. His mother made arrangements to spend the night on the floor."

"What was the problem?" Jerry asked.

"I'll get to that. On Monday when I tried to examine Sam, I was struck that he was a disturbed little boy. There was a tremor of his hands, and when I moved toward him, he pulled the sheet up to his neck," Rick said. "It took four days to find out what the problem was. Sam had a friend named Jacob. The boys were on the same schedule, so last fall, they were on the floor the same week getting POMP. Jacob relapsed in January and received a second course of daunomycin in February. In March, Jacob was terminally ill, and Sam spent a lot of time in Jacob's room. Sam was discharged on Friday, and Jacob died the next week."

"When Sam returned to 2 East in April, he asked Barbara where Jacob was, and she told him Jacob had been transferred to 12 East," Rick said.

Jerry and I sat in silence. I felt pain for Sam. I felt sorry that Barbara's good intentions had turned out so wrong. Barbara was dedicated to the children of 2 East. I thought, children could handle the diagnosis of leukemia. Explicit disclosure of death was not yet part of being honest with children. Tommy and his question about heaven had taught me that kids know about death: Jon wanted to know if a green sign was hung on his door, and children paraded up and down the hall trying to look into the room of a dying child—they all knew about death, even if moms, nurses, and doctors didn't tell them.

In July, Sam would be transferred to his own 12 East.

• • •

On Sunday nights, I often drove into Bethesda for an Italian dinner or Maryland steamed crabs. Then I would look in on 2 East to see if there were any admissions for chemotherapy the next day. Some moms preferred to come in then rather than battle Monday-morning traffic. I liked doing the interim history and physical and writing my admission notes on that evening; it was one less thing for me to do the next morning. The pace was more relaxed. It was an opportunity to talk to the child and mother. Often Jerry and almost always Rick came in then.

It was on one of these occasions that I found a four-year-old boy in the middle of the hall, crying and screaming. "His name is Fred," Barbara explained. "Fred is generally dropped off on Sunday night; his mom has to work. When his mother leaves, he has a temper tantrum. Candy, ice cream, or being held doesn't help, so we just let Fred cry for half an hour, and then he's OK."

I sat down on the floor, picked up Fred, and placed him on my lap. That only increased the screaming, and he hit me on the chest. I looked up to find Rick standing over the two of us.

"Ben, you can't console a toddler who feels abandoned. That's Fred; we go through this every month."

Eventually, Fred's hitting and screaming gave way to crying and deep sobs. "I know," I said. "I don't have anything better to do."

"Ben, if I ever met anyone who should go into pediatrics, it's you." Rick meant it as a compliment.

• • •

One evening in late May, Frank came into the kitchen where I was reading a journal and announced, "I'm getting married next month."

"Congratulations! Tell me about it."

Information, excitement, and plans flowed, as Frank unfolded several months of planning for a wedding.

I just listened, and I was pleased to learn that much of the time he wasn't here on weekends and nights had been spent dating and not working in the lab.

An hour passed, as a good friend shared good news with me.

JUNE

Only one month left. Time to say good-bye to the children, their mothers, and the nurses of 2 East. I needed closure. I had never experienced anything like this before. At the end of a three-month rotation during my residency in medicine, there was only a question of "What's next?" For eleven months, I had watched how courageously children dealt with adversity. I stuck needles in them, and they, in return, shared their world with me. For the next four weeks, I'd walk onto 2 East, but it wasn't the same 2 East I'd entered eleven months ago, and I wasn't the same person.

• • •

Saying good-bye wasn't always possible or even desirable.

On Tuesday morning, the first week of June, Rick asked, "Did you know Morgan resigned last week?"

"I thought she was on vacation," Jerry said.

Almost a year before, Morgan had shown me around and introduced me to what I called my patients on that first day of July. "Did we miss a farewell party? I would have liked to thank her, wished her well, said good-bye. Did she transfer to another unit?"

Rick shrugged. "She went back to Boston where she trained. Dee told me most of the nurses don't want a good-bye party."

"That's odd."

"Think about it, Ben," Jerry said. "At the end of this month, we're going to leave. Do you want a party with a cake that reads, 'Thank You, Dr. Humphrey'? Do you want Dee to make a little speech? Or Jay? Do we want a party for all three of us, 'Thank You, Doctors,' written all over a cake?"

"No," I said. "Not at all."

Rick shook his head, and Jerry added, "Neither do I."

• • •

Mrs. Shively called me to ask if Carl could be seen in the clinic. "Is Carl all right?'

"Oh yes," she said, "I know we're not due for a clinic appointment until July. I hope you don't mind seeing us a little early. We're going to Paris."

Relieved, I said, "It would be a pleasure to see you before you leave on vacation,"—a formal, sterile response. For Carl's mom, I could have said, "Hell yes. Come on in."

Mrs. Shively arrived in a full gale of bluster. Not without reason, she wanted Carl to have a bone-marrow aspirate, as she said, "Just to make sure we don't have to rush home."

While waiting for the marrow to be processed, I called Myron Karon and asked, "Do you know an oncologist in Paris?"

Having spent a year there, Myron did know one who spoke English. "Georges Mathé in Villejuif, south of Paris. He's good but a bit on the wild side. Do you think your patient's mom can handle an outgoing physician?"

The question was more likely to be, could Doctor Mathé handle Mrs. Shively?

After giving Carl and his mother the good news about his marrow, I gave Mrs. Shively the doctor's name and address.

I learned that she had majored in art at Georgetown and spent a year there. As usual, Mrs. Shively was full of surprises.

"I assumed you were a college graduate because you used *catharsis* during Carl's visit in March."

"You remember that. Well, I'm not surprised. You're bright."

To keep this routine going, I told her, "We're trying to find a clinical associate for next year who has only one head."

"I did say that back in October, didn't I? We're going to miss you, Doc, but I guess a year for you guys on 2 East is enough for anybody."

Good old Mrs. Shively. Lucky Carl and I shook hands, and Mrs. Shively gave me a big hug. I thought, I'll recall bits and fragments of conversations from every mother I've come in contact with this year, but I'll probably go to my grave remembering every wonderful word Mrs. Shively ever said.

● ● ●

Robert 'Gosh' Thurman had some more pictures and stories of Sparky to show me, now part of our routine.

"Best thing that has come into our home since Robert was born," Mr. Thurman said. "We thought we were doing this for Robert, but Sparky has been good for all of us."

"That's great."

Todd, Mrs. Yardley, and Ralph came to mind, but I let the thought pass.

When Robert asked if Polly had been admitted, I told him I didn't think so, but he could go ask the nurses. Robert hopped off the bed and was out the door.

Mr. Thurman smiled. "They're an odd pair. They often pat each other on their bald heads. Polly likes to play the older sister, and I think Robert has a crush on her. His first girlfriend."

"Your son has good taste in women."

When Robert returned, I promised to send her to see him so they could visit for awhile before the bone marrows.

Brigid and I were in the hall when we heard, "Hey, Doc, I got something to show you." Polly came bouncing down the hall, her mother in hot pursuit. "Get a load of this T-shirt."

When Mrs. Sorensen said it would be better to show me in the room, Polly said, "I want to show the shirt to Brigid too." Polly undid the braces of her denim overalls and let the bib drop. In bold black letters against bright blue was printed:

**I'm bald
and beautiful
and Dr. H is my barber.**

Brigid and I laughed; I had to wipe a tear away. "Go down to room seven and show Robert Thurman," I said. "He's been asking to see you."

"I hope you're not offended, Doctor Humphrey. Last weekend we were in Rehoboth Beach, and Polly got this idea as we walked by a shop that advertised made-to-order T-shirts. I didn't think it was appropriate, but her father thought it would be OK. Polly has that man wrapped around her little finger."

"I'm wrapped around that same finger, Mrs. Sorensen," I said.

Brigid added, "Me, too."

• • •

Jay gave our last seminar. The lecture was easy to follow, very detailed, and included an analysis of VAMP, BIKE, and POMP. Jay's first graph stressed the poor prognosis of children who did not achieve a remission with the first course of therapy. Table after table followed with clinical trials by NIH and other institutes.

Of special interest was the data from NIH on unmaintained remission. There were kids off therapy; a few had relapsed, but most were in remission. Jay was cautious when he said, "The evidence suggests we are curing fifteen percent of children with ALL, but I want to follow these kids for a few more years."

Back to the floor, Rick said, "I hope it's true, but after a year on 2 East, it's hard to see fifteen percent."

• • •

"Ben, can we go feed your squirrel?" Jerry asked. His voice was low. "I even bought a bag of peanuts."

Jerry commented on the pleasant weather in the way one does when trying to fill a void. We sat down. I was in no hurry and let Jerry take his time. Son of Squirrel finally saw us and descended.

"Remember Joan Loken, my five-year-old, the one with the big blue bunny rabbit who died in March?"

"Yes, the rabbit was almost as big as Joan."

"Well, her mother came in yesterday just to be on 2 East again. Of course she was welcome, but I was surprised how much I enjoyed listening to her talk about Joan."

What was haunting Jerry was the way Mrs. Loken talked as if Joan were still alive, now just someplace else. "She might have meant heaven, but she didn't refer to heaven," Jerry said. "Her visit to 2 East helped her connect to her daughter."

"I like it when the parents of a dead child return to 2 East," I said.

"Ben, do you remember when we went for coffee and talked about poetry, plays, and that sort of stuff? We both said we liked Thornton Wilder. Well, yesterday was a day for *The Bridge of San Luis Rey*."

"You don't have to memorize the end of the novel; it just sticks to you: 'There's the land of the dead and the land of the living, and the bridge between them is love,'" I said.

"That's almost a direct quote," Jerry said. "I was so haunted by Wilder's novel that I stopped by the library in Georgetown, pulled a copy off the shelf, sat down just to flip through a few pages, and ended up checking it out of the library."

"Mrs. Loken may not have read *The Bridge of San Luis Rey*, but she sure is in contact with the essence of that novel," Jerry said.

• • •

Hilary O'Keefe, my gentle Irish rose, came in for her monthly POMP. Vincristine had taken its toll, and all the brownish-red hair was gone but not the pleasant gaze. I sat on the bed and held out my hand, and she laid hers in mine.

"Hilary, you continue to respond to therapy. Your bone marrow is full of good cells—no bad cells."

"All the mothers know that the three of you will be leaving 2 East at the end of the week," Mrs. O'Keefe said. "I can only imagine that you all are eager to get on with your next assignment. We're going to miss all three of you, but we wish you well."

I sat back. Here was a mother very involved in her daughter's care, yet able to sense how the three of us might feel. I admitted, "It's been a long year."

"Ma," Hilary said, extending her hand toward her mother.

"Here you are, dear," Mrs. O'Keefe said as she handed her daughter a photo.

"It's for you," Hilary smiled.

It was a two-and-a-half-by-three-and-a-half-inch black-and-white photo of Hilary sitting at a table, her arms folded in front of her, her head tilted to the left, her eyes gazing to the left, wearing one of those smiles a child can flash when she knows her picture is about to be taken.

"Thank you, Hilary, it's a very nice picture."
That was in 1965, a gift from a cherub; I still have the photo.

• • •

I was aware of a subtle dilemma, especially on this Friday. My responsibilities would be over in less than a week, but my next assignment was right there in the Clinical Center. I could just stop by and say hello, to the nurses, to the moms, and to my children. But did I really want to be there on the week when a child relapsed or was being treated for sepsis? Despite Jay's prediction of disease-free survival, my assumption was that all the children would die. Did I need to know when?

I remember trying to resolve this dilemma on the basis of the transfer of responsibility. The moms needed to look to the new associates, learn to trust these individuals, and not be tempted to ask for a different opinion from one of last year's associates. I thought of that first day in July. It never occurred to me that Billingsworth would return to 2 East. Why would my replacement want me to return?

This wasn't a time to figure things out; this was a moment for saying good-bye.

I returned to Hilary's room and said an awkward farewell to this very special child. However, there was a trade-off. I might never again see her wonderful smile, but I would never again have to hurt her.

• • •

That night at the fence an intuition came to me, and I recognized it as an epiphany. I'd been given a photo of Hilary, a little girl whom Jay Freireich was trying to cure. That might not happen, but she would live a little longer. Her life would be extended. That was what was important.

The seed of this reality had been planted by Mrs. Paul in September when she said to me, "You know, Doctor, when your child is four years old, four months is a lot of time." A calmness settled over me that was temporarily broken by a few indignant thoughts about the assholes of academic medicine who criticized Sidney Farber at Harvard who used methotrexate to put kids into short-lived remissions and those who now criticized Jay Freireich and Tom Frei for trying to cure children. These negative thoughts were quickly dismissed as images of one child after another came to me, children who had enriched my life, children whom I had had the privilege of knowing. Medicine can't after all prevent death, but it can extend life.

It was time for a sound night's sleep.

• • •

"I've got a great picture of my son," Rick said as he added another frame to the collection on his desk. In the photo, Erik was propped in the sitting position by a pillow and wearing a suit with bow tie and a smile.

"He's cute, and that's a nice outfit," Jerry said.

"Yeah," Rick said proudly. "It fits, and the colors match. Jody picked out the suit, and I chose the bow tie."

"Why wouldn't it fit?" I asked.

"When I was training in Seattle and Minneapolis, some of the residents were raising infants or even toddlers. Most of the kids' clothes came from Goodwill and were often too large or had colors that didn't match."

"Yeah, I can imagine raising a kid is expensive," Jerry added.

"Not when you're being paid a lieutenant commander's salary. Jody and I never think twice about buying things for Erik."

I chuckled. "I never think about money here on the East Coast until I walk into a bookstore and buy a new unused book. I get exactly the book, I want, and if they don't have it, they'll order a copy for me, and

I'll pay full price. What a change. All of my adult years used to be spent in secondhand bookstores."

"Well, I don't have to look at my checkbook before I go out to dinner, and I'm eating in fine restaurants. At Christmas, I flew up to Maine to see my parents and didn't give a thought to the cost."

We all agreed: we now looked at our checking balance once a month instead of daily.

• • •

Monday, and the names of Dan "Supportive" Martin and Billy "Bear" Sullivan were on the Board. Dee introduced me to Elaine, a new face, who was considering joining the nursing staff.

Elaine was five ten and thin. Her black hair was cut pageboy style, and the frames of her oval glasses were tinted rose. She seemed at ease, following the conversation between Dee and me by looking directly at each of us.

Dee had worked out a schedule so that Elaine could observe all that went into a Monday morning. Elaine accompanied me as I made my rounds. Before obtaining an interim history and doing the monthly examination of Dan Martin and Billy Sullivan, I explained the difference in coping styles of the two mothers. In the treatment room, I went through the procedure of breaking the bone. During the aspirations, Elaine held each of the boys, Dee standing directly behind her. I took the marrow sample up to pathology, and Dee and Elaine joined Jerry, who had only one admission. Billy and Dan were both in remission. While I started the IVs, Elaine held both boys. She reassured them in a calm voice. After an IV was established, the slight frown on her forehead disappeared, and she told Billy, "Well, we're both glad that's over." Billy rewarded her with a smile, which she returned.

I saw Dee working alone in her office and had to ask, "How do you find nurses for 2 East? How did you know to hire Morgan and Brigid?"

"When I first started working as head nurse, I thought I knew what was important—even had some criteria to use during an interview. But nothing seems to correlate with a nurse staying on the job for a year or more. Some candidates are idealistic, and others are very concerned that they might not be able to control their emotions. Some are tired of a high-volume pediatric practice where all they do is give shots. Some had a relative or a friend who died of cancer—on and on the reasons go. I'm of the opinion that none of that helps to predict who's going to do well."

Rick's comment that nothing prepares one for the children of 2 East flashed through my mind. "Having them spend Monday morning on 2 East is a good idea."

"Yeah, it gives a young nurse an opportunity to back out gracefully," Dee explained. "You know, we tell 'em to observe first and then think it over. There're a couple of other things. If at the end of the morning a candidate is still interested, I have one of the staff take the candidate out to lunch, someplace off campus. I tell my staff, 'Don't tell 'em it's a great job. Just listen, answer their questions, and ask yourself, is this someone I'd like to work with?' I'm more interested in their opinions than my own."

"If after a morning on 2 East the candidate orders three martinis before lunch, that's not a good sign."

We laughed.

• • •

Frank had finished his two years in the laboratory in Bethesda. Even before starting his tour of duty at NIH, Frank knew he'd be returning to the University of Chicago, where he'd taken his residency in pediatrics. He was bright, a very good clinician, and the chairman of pediatrics wanted him to return to join the faculty when he finished his military service.

Frank's transient venture into the world of being an equestrian now over, he sold Galla-B to Mindy. When she picked up the Thoroughbred, she asked, "Have you been thrown yet, Ben?"

"Oh yes."

"I knew you were going to be a quick learner."

Domino wasn't sold. Frank's mother had found a farm where Domino could graze at his leisure; Frank could visit on trips to see his mother. I liked that. Domino wasn't a horse: he was a pet. I knew I'd miss the evening routine of carrots, the reflections on life at the fence, and those occasional bareback rides.

Shonto of course would be going to Chicago. Black labs tend to do well wherever they are. I wondered if dogs could reminisce. Would Shonto miss the horses' water tank and those thrilling days of baiting Domino and jumping to safety in the nick of time? I knew I would miss the cold, wet nose that occasionally woke me on weekends when I tried to sleep in.

Frank was married in June. He and his bride, Nina, would be heading for Chicago at the end of the month. Frank had a future.

Fortunately the Kirkhill idyll would last another year for me. I had no plans to look for a roommate. In fact, I had no plans for the future. A lot of things were coming to an end.

• • •

During my last week on 2 East, Dee told me Mrs. Graham wanted to visit the floor and if possible stop by to say hello. At two in the afternoon, Dee opened the office door for Mrs. Graham. Gone were the dark circles from under her eyes; she appeared to have regained some weight, but I had the impression that she was years older than the mother I had met a year ago.

"Good afternoon, Mrs. Graham. Won't you please sit down?"

"Hi, Doctor Humphrey. I won't take too much of your time."

"Mrs. Graham, I have lots of time. I'm very pleased to see you again."

"I was just talking to the nurses. I am sorry to learn Morgan is no longer here. When things were running smoothly, she had a peppy, upbeat manner of caring for John. When she puffed up his pillow, she'd tell him it was a government regulation—all children must rest their heads on soft pillows."

I sat back in my chair and crossed my legs, and the two of us exchanged memories of John. We talked about when we met and the attempt to use art to help John. Mrs. Graham also told me of the other mothers she was in contact with.

When I asked how John's father was doing, she said that was one reason she wanted to see me. "John Sr. has always been a good family man and a great father. The first two or three months after John's death were absolute hell for me. I don't think I could have gotten through February and March without his support...Of course he was going through the same hell." She went into some detail about their life in April and May and how things were now different. "I know I'll always be the mother of John, our son, who died here on 2 East. Out of this experience, I—no, we—my husband and I have been given something. *Given* is not quite the right word. At any rate, we're different." She stopped and smiled. "John Sr. wanted me to share all that with you and the nurses."

"You're 'different.' Tell me about that."

"Well, let me start with February. Any thought about my son right after his death caused sleepless nights—inconsolable crying. I still cry, but now my tears are an expression of the loss—like it's OK for me to have sorrow." She paused. "That may not make sense. Let me give you another example. Little things, things of no real consequence, are less likely to be seen as major events. John Sr. can be very impatient when mechanical things don't work. Two weeks ago the car wouldn't start. His only reaction was, 'I'll check the battery, and if that's not it, we'll have it towed to the garage and rent a car until it's fixed.' I couldn't believe it. And when he saw me smiling, he shrugged and said, 'It's not the worst thing that's ever happened to us.'"

"No resentment over the car."

"Ah, there's an important word—*resentment*," Mrs. Graham said. "Right after John's death, my best friend told me she knew how I felt. I was indignant. How dare she presume to know? I didn't want to ever see her again. Now when she tries to be my companion in grief, I know she means well. I know she wants to help, and that's what's important."

All I could do was nod.

"Let me give you another example," Mrs. Graham said. "My sister and I took her four-year-old for ice cream. Crossing a busy street, I took his hand. That would have been just to keep him safe. But when it happened, I recognized how small and warm his hand was and how I was again touching a child." Tears rolled down her cheeks.

I was at a loss. Finally I said, "John was your son. That's got to be special. On 2 East, I hear the staff, the nurses, and the doctors referring to 'our children,' or 'one of my children'—things like that."

Mrs. Graham interrupted me with a big smile. "Morgan would do that. After she'd take John's temperature, she'd put her hands on her hips and say, 'John! Of all my children here on 2 East, you're the most difficult to get a smile from. Now come on, John.' Sometimes she could tease one out of him."

I walked her to the front door and thanked her for coming in. Watching her leave, I thought, she looks older, but you too are older, much older than just from the passing of a year.

Walking over to my bench, I was greeted by Son of Squirrel. "I miss your dad, but I'm glad I've got you. You know, little buddy, I guess I'll always be a doctor who spent a year on 2 East, and it took a mother to help me recognize that I too have been given something. Mrs. Graham will always have to deal with the legacy of grief, and I'll have to deal with a different kind of legacy. It'll take a while for me to figure out what I've been given."

● ● ●

G. Bennett Humphrey

Tuesday afternoon, June 29. Time to clean out my desk, empty the drawers, and select what to keep and what to throw away.

From the lower-right-hand file drawer, I pulled out multiple folders, hand labeled, containing photocopies of articles on problems in leukemia and clinical trials related to pediatrics and pediatric oncology. As an internist I should have just chucked them. To someone who would be working in a biochemistry lab next year, none of these were of any value. I put them in a cardboard box—something to sort out on a rainy day.

The upper-right-hand drawer was simple. I chucked the ballpoint pens that didn't work, the three-by-five cards I hadn't used, and the dried-up yellow highlighter. A couple of bags of peanuts went in my pocket; there might be problems in biochemistry I would need to share with Son of Squirrel. I wasn't smart enough to know what the bigger questions would be: What's the plan for the years after NIH? What the hell am I going to do with the rest of my life?

Looking at this desk of one year, I remembered my feelings about emptying my eight-year desk in the laboratory at the University of Chicago. It was also a June day just before commencement when I received my PhD and a couple of weeks prior to leaving for Germany. That was a desk of accomplishments, where I had studied the preclinical disciplines of pathology, microbiology, and all those other -ologies; wrote up my case presentations for medicine, surgery, and pediatrics while classical music played in the background; crammed for three months for my preliminary exam in biochemistry; learned enough French and German to pass the language requirements for a PhD; prepared my PhD thesis; and, most midnights, listened to the sign-off poem from WFMT. I recognized that I had been sad but also excited and had looked forward to my year in Germany.

I didn't dislike this NIH desk. It had been a good work area, but it wasn't associated with anything I recognized as an accomplishment: a place where every Monday morning I read the *New York Times* to remind me that mine was not the only war, a space to write notes into the charts of my children and where there had been no radio, no music, and no recordings of poets reading their poems.

After closing the drawers, I picked up my yellow pad. The first column listed names. In between the second column, "Date of Diagnosis" and the fourth, "Miscellaneous Data," was the third column, "Date of Death." Sitting back in my chair, I read of Baby Boy William, who had never been held by his mother. Jimmy Paul, who wanted to know how kids got into heaven, Jeff Donaldson, who charmed us all in his quiet way, Tammy Long, my pied beauty, and Penny Tapley, who defended her personal space to the end. Todd Yardley with his tales of Ralph, and Michelle Karr, a snuggle bunny for my lap. Images of each child came to me as I read the names, feeling indescribably hollow.

• • •

Wednesday at 2:37 p.m., Rick suggested, "Let's go for coffee." Down in the cafeteria, we sat together for the last time as clinical associates of 2 East. The conversation was halting and reflective.

"You guys have done very well, you know—well, for internists on a pediatric unit." Rick smiled. "On the first of July, I thought I knew it all; I mean, I'd had a two-year fellowship in pediatric hem-onc." He looked down and stirred his coffee. "It didn't take me long to find out I wasn't prepared for 2 East."

No one said anything.

"I remember the first time you told me that, Rick," I said. "It blew me away."

"Well, Ben, we always knew Rick was there, ready to throw either of us a lifeline," Jerry said. "It was the nurses that astonished me. I'd think, I'm here on 2 East because I don't want to be in Vietnam. Then I'd see a nurse help a child, and I'd think, she's here because she wants to be, wants to serve." He looked down at his cup. "It often made me feel very small."

I thought about Jerry's remark.

"Let me share something with you two," I said. "I was eased into adult medicine; as a junior and senior med student, I watched, as an intern, I worked, and as a resident, I supervised. For five years, I was a member of a team seeing adults, and during all those years, I never thought of my childhood. A year ago, I found myself in a room with a child and his mother. Later, I realized kids were sharing their childhood with me, and I started to search my own stories to share with them. A wild, wild experience—an unforgettable voyage—with good shipmates."

"A boat ride over smooth waters and turbulent seas," Jerry said.

The conversation was a bit sentimental. We were looking at one another, when Rick said, "Hey, we'll be seeing each other all next year."

True, but it wouldn't be the same. The days of *Drie Kameraden* were over.

• • •

Saying good-bye was over. I had indirectly been saying good-bye to dying children starting out on the first week with Baby Boy Williams. During the last few weeks, I had said good-bye to children still alive. I wasn't very good at it.

Thursday morning, I awoke early. Chores were simple; Whirley-Wee was the only horse to feed. I thought of Shonto as I filled the water trough; I missed her not being part of my morning.

When I arrived on 2 East, Rick was already on the floor, and Jerry joined us soon thereafter. All the IVs were running. The new clinical associates were in a one-hour orientation lecture.

The three of us sat in the office. We didn't have much to talk about. There was the assumption that we'd see each other now and then here in the Clinical Center. Rick's laboratory was just down the hall from mine, and Jerry would be working two floors above.

We didn't plan on going to lunch or for cocktails and dinner. There was nothing to celebrate.

My replacement was a tall guy from Ohio. An internist. I don't remember his name. I would be more cordial than Billingsworth had been with me. I would spend as much time with him as he wished. After a few exchanges, he said he wanted to start and didn't feel it was necessary for me to introduce him to, as he put it, "my new patients."

I wished him well. As I walked off 2 East, I thought, they're not patients; they're children.

Epilogue

Summer

As if in a posttraumatic daze, July and August passed. In the morning, I enjoyed watching Whirley-Wee trot up to the fence. She didn't have to race up to her hay and oats because there was no competition.

I went to my assigned research laboratory at nine. The director of the lab was a delightful MD, PhD from Harvard. He was quiet by nature and very scholarly in his approach to research. He also played the cello.

I didn't spend any time looking for a place where I could complete my third year of residency in medicine or where I should apply for a two-year fellowship in hematology.

In the evening, I often worked with Whirley-Wee and enjoyed the beauty and power of her gaits. At twilight, I only brought a carrot to the fence: no problems and no disturbed emotions.

In late August, Rick walked into my laboratory and told me, "Ben, come on down to my lab. I've got my boss, Bill Krivit, on the phone. I've told him about you, and he wants to invite you to come to Minnesota and give a talk on the research you did in Germany. I've told him I think you ought to go into pediatrics."

Having a prepared talk might come in handy and get me back into thinking about my future.

Three weeks later, I walked into Rick's laboratory and told him, "I guess my seminar in Minneapolis went well. Krivit offered me a position, and I accepted."

It was a pivotal moment. The children had worked their magic on me, and I was pleased to acknowledge that fact. The truth was I was now looking forward to the future.

Rick shook my hand and flashed that wonderful smile of his. Now it was a smile of "Welcome aboard."

The End

Acknowledgments

During the past few years, I have made the acquaintance of more than a score of writers. Many have become friends, and all these individuals have provided me with valuable comments.

Special kudos to three writers who read multiple drafts of my manuscript and provided me with valuable support and commentary throughout the development of the book: Annie Dawid, Patricia Nolan, and Summer Wood.

I very much appreciate Doctor Gerald (Jerry) Sandler and Doctor Emil J. (Jay) Freireich, who took time from their professional responsibilities to read and approve the contents of a very lengthy draft of the manuscript.

All projects of this type begin somewhere, and I was fortunate to be a member of the San Luis Valley Literary Society, whose members encouraged me to pursue this subject: Rhonda Boarders, Francie Hall, and Mary Lampe.

The following individuals read sections of various lengths from early drafts: Peggy Godfrey, and from James McKean's workshop at the 2012 Iowa Summer Writing Festival, Sue Bonner, Karen Gershowitz, Pickens Halt, and Mary Mellon.

My Taos master class 2013 fellow students were: Bonnie Alexander, Mary Beth, Mathew Binder, Frances Burke, and Carolyn Flynn. Summer Wood conducted the class and these individuals read a very long version of my ms.

G. Bennett Humphrey

University of New Mexico's Taos master class 2014 was conducted by Justin St. Germain and the following writers who were accepted into the workshop: Kaatje van der Gaarden, Mishele Maron, and Brian Wolf. These individuals critiqued a shorter draft of my ms.

The fine-tuning of later drafts of this manuscript was accomplished with the help of Rita O'Connell, Pickens Halt, and Cynthia Storrs.

Again, special thanks to Doctor Sandler, who read the final draft of my manuscript and provided me with the foreword to the book.

I have enjoyed working on this manuscript. Recalling and writing about my year on 2 East often brought tears of happiness and sorrow, which I gladly shed. Not a release of tension, writing *Breaking Little Bones* has been a journey of spiritual joy, an opportunity to share with the reader the many experiences of one year of my life.

G. Bennett (Ben) Humphrey
Boulder and Fort Garland, Colorado July 2016

Commentaries from NIH colleagues of 1964

"The children of 2 East. A moving recall of a young physician on the battlefront of the effort to develop curative therapy for a systemic cancer, acute leukemia in children. Highly readable and descriptive. The reader will be transported to 2 East of 1964. Ben tells it like it was in the 1960s. I loved his book even though he called me a schmuck.'"

Emil J. Freireich, MD, internationally recognized research oncologist, and the supervisor to 2 East and the author as a clinical associate

"I started to read it and could not put it down. Dr. Humphrey has a very readable style—direct, quick, and clear. He captures the sense of 2 East."

Gerald S. Sandler, MD, friend from 2 East, long and successful academic career at Georgetown University

"I finished your manuscript. A lot of work and skilled, careful polishing— also a sad memorial to all those brave children who gave their lives eventually to save others."

Frank K. Thorp, MD, PhD, friend, roommate at Kirkhill Farm, and later, an academic pediatrician specializing in diabetes

Author's note

The names of the following physicians or scientists have not been altered: Emil J. (Jay) Freireich, Emil (Tom) Frie, Myron Karon, Gerald S. (Jerry) Sandler, Fredrick (Rick) Lottsfeldt, Frank K. Thorp, and Eugene Goldwasser,

Doctors Freireich, Sandler, and Thorp have read and endorsed the ideas present in this book.

Unfortunately, the rest of the individuals listed above are dead. Doctor Lottsfeldt died after an automobile accident in 1966, a few months before he was to move back to Seattle and start his academic career at the University of Washington Medical School. Doctor Karon's fatal stroke in 1974 was also an early death.

The rest of the individuals described are real people, but their names, certain identifying characteristics, and temporal events have been changed. Many of the children and a few of the mothers are composites.

After 2 East, my own personal future included marriage and fatherhood.

About the Author

G. Bennett Humphrey, MD, PhD, completed his graduate studies in medicine and biochemistry at the University of Chicago. Following the events of this book, he retrained in pediatrics, with oncology and hematology as his subspecialties. He taught pediatric oncology at a number of universities, including as a visiting professor in Japan, Europe, and the United States.

Over his career Humphrey has written numerous articles and chapters and has edited several pediatric oncology books. In 2013 his chapbook entitled *The Magpie Cried*, containing poems about his youth, was published. That year he was named Senior Poet Laureate of Colorado. Three short stories from this book have been published previously, two by Whispering Angel Press and the other by Johns Hopkins University Press. Humphrey currently splits time between his apartment in Boulder, Colorado, and a cabin in the Sangre de Cristo Mountains at ninety-three hundred feet, just north of the New Mexico border.